To Danielle Love Mum x

EATING FOR A
PERFECT PREGNANCY

This Book Belongs 2005
to Ruth

GM00802489

30130 116306654

Also by Suzannah Olivier

. . . .

What Should I Feed My Baby?

The Breast Cancer Prevention and Recovery Diet

The Stress Protection Plan

Also by Suzannah Olivier in the *You Are What You Eat* series

. . . .

Banish Bloating

Maximising Energy

Natural Hormone Balance

The Detox Manual

Allergy Solutions

Suzannah Olivier

EATING FOR

A PERFECT

PREGNANCY

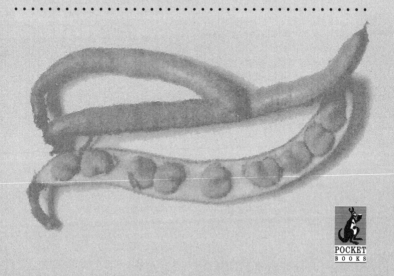

POCKET
B O O K S

For the next generation: Benedict, Sam, Phoebe and Isaac

Thanks to Julie Packer of the Portland Hospital for all her invaluable help

First published in Great Britain by Pocket Books, 2001
An imprint of Simon & Schuster UK Ltd
A Viacom Company

10 9 8 7 6 5 4 3 2 1

Simon & Schuster UK Ltd
Africa House
64-78 Kingsway
London WC2B 6AH

Simon & Schuster Australia
Sydney

A CIP catalogue record for this book is available from the British Library

ISBN 0-671-03781-1

My aim in writing this book was to gather together the best knowledge
currently available on nutrition during pregnancy. It is not intended as an
alternative to the advice you receive from your doctor or midwife.
If you are in any doubt about any symptoms you must consult your
medical advisers.

Typeset in 12 on 14pt Perpetua with Gill Sans display
Design and page make-up by Peter Ward
Printed and bound in Great Britain by Omnia Books Limited, Glasgow

Contents

PART FOUR

NOW YOU ARE A PARENT

PART FIVE

RESOURCES

Part One

PREPARING FOR
A PERFECT
PREGNANCY

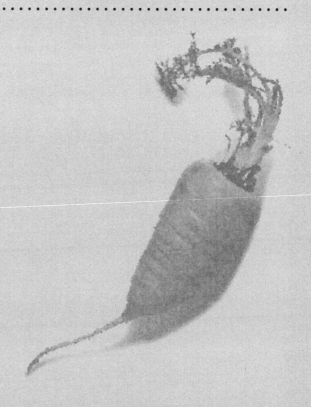

Introduction

What is 'Eating for a Perfect Pregnancy'? In essence, it involves making sure that every mouthful of food you eat is a power-packed source of nourishment, enabling you to grow the healthiest possible baby. All food is not equal, and all calories are not equal. Some foods give you a superb range of nutrients that your body can use to build optimal health, while others not only fail to provide these nutrients, but also prevent you from using the nutrients you do get properly. Nowadays many people are well fed, and yet at the same time undernourished.

While the benefits of nutrition continue to be controversial in some areas of health care, there is one area where its importance is virtually unchallenged. Optimal nutrition before, and during pregnancy, indisputably leads to healthier babies, and to healthier mothers. A pivotal study at The Harvard School of Public Health showed that women who had the best diets had a 95 per cent chance of having a baby in superb health. This was compared to women who had average diets, 88 per cent of whose babies were in fair/good health and only 6 per cent of whom had babies in first rate health. At the bottom end of the scale only 8 per cent of women who had diets that consisted largely of junk food had babies who were in good or excellent health, and 65 per cent of these women had babies who were stillborn, premature, functionally immature or born with congenital defects. Other studies have since backed up these findings.

Certainly, in the West, now is a very good time indeed to be born. Developments in the field of obstetrics, and in antenatal and postnatal care, have improved the outcomes for babies and mothers in a way almost unrivalled in any other field of medicine. The infant mortality rate has been slashed to levels only dreamed of previously; better infant and maternal care has ensured that babies who are born pre-term have an increasingly good chance of survival; couples who have a history of fertility or pregnancy problems are nursed through all the options to improve their chances of having a family.

THE NUTRITION LINK

However, despite the fantastic advances made in obstetric care in the last century, we should not be too quick to pat ourselves on the back. It may astound you to learn that in a 1998 survey of underweight babies covering 35 countries the UK appeared near the bottom, and ranked only just ahead of Hungary, Bulgaria, Romania and Turkey. Even Albania and Latvia, where they do not have access to such sophisticated medical facilities as we do, had better records than ours. What is the reason for this? Almost certainly it is related to nutrition, and to exposure to alcohol, smoking and other womb pollutants during pregnancy. The diets of many people in the UK are worryingly deficient in the basic nutrients: 31 per cent of women have diets deficient in vitamin A, 47 per cent are low in folic acid, 34 per cent do not get enough vitamin C, 48 per cent are deficient in calcium, 32 per cent need more iodine, a whopping 89 per cent are low in iron, while 72 per cent lack magnesium and 31 per cent are zinc paupers. This is not conducive to producing the healthiest babies.

If we are to see any further advances in the reduction of pregnancy and childbirth risks it is likely to need the active participation of expectant parents. Expectant mothers – and expectant fathers – will need to prepare for pregnancy far more than they do now, by addressing, for example, deficiencies in their diet and lifestyle. Pre-pregnancy checks, such as screening for infections, will also need to become routine. Of course, the medicalisation of pregnancy and childbirth can only work up to a point. These are, after all, natural events, not illnesses, and yet focusing on preventive care and the best nutrition practices before and during your pregnancy will help you avoid being a 'patient' and give your baby the best start in life.

The main aim of this book is to ensure that you, your baby and your partner are nourished as well as possible prior to, during and after your pregnancy, so that you feel fit and energetic despite your changing body and the inevitable interrupted sleep that follows after you have your baby. If you are determined to make the best of your pregnancy and have the healthiest possible baby to cuddle, enjoy, tickle and hug, then give yourself, and your baby, the best chance by eating and drinking for optimal health.

It is a bit of a minefield out there and you cannot take for granted that everything is 'safe' and you really do need to learn to look out for yourself and your baby. The cynical way that food giants treat the future generation, even when they are in the womb, came home to me with huge impact when I received a promotional package of 'gifts' at my antenatal classes. In the pack was a leaflet, on the cover of which was a picture of various healthy foods (orange juice, grapes, wholemeal bread, etc) with the slogan 'Now, more than ever, you are being careful about what you eat and drink'. Inside was a picture of a beautiful mother and baby with another line about wanting to avoid caffeine. Finally on the last spread was the real advertisement – for a caffeine free, artificially sweetened leading brand of cola. The fact that this product could be specifically marketed to pregnant women is one of the major incentives for writing this book.

HOW TO USE THIS BOOK

This book begins with a chapter on pre-pregnancy planning, which is followed by ones on eating during pregnancy, solutions to common problems during each of the three trimesters, and, finally, the time just after the delivery. I imagine, however, that many people reading this book will already be pregnant. If that is the case with you, you can turn first to **Eating for a Perfect Pregnancy** (page 49). However, much of the information in the previous chapter, **Preparing for a Perfect Pregnancy**, will still be relevant to you, including that on infections, medicines, vitamin and mineral supplements and alcohol, so you'd be wise to read that too. When you reach the chapter on solutions to common problems, don't be daunted by the long list of possible complaints. You will not get all of them, and hopefully, by following the dietary advice, you will not get any. Even if you do, you have the means to deal with them, and in any event amnesia sets in afterwards – if it didn't the future of the human race would be in doubt!

CHAPTER ONE

Preparing for a Perfect Pregnancy

In an ideal world both partners would plan for pregnancy at least three months, and preferably six months, before conception. Of course this is not always possible. 'Surprises' often happen – and thank goodness they do. Wouldn't it be dull if we always planned everything? But for those in a stable relationship, who know they want to start a family, it is wise to start thinking about the health of both parents-to-be in order to optimise the chances of a healthy pregnancy.

Even if you are able to plan ahead, do not be disappointed if you do not manage to conceive when you intend to – nature is fickle indeed. Nevertheless there is much that can be done to increase the likelihood of fertility, as we will see later.

MAKING BABIES

Your baby is made, purely and simply, of the raw materials that you provide: a healthy egg and sperm, nourishment to develop, and a safe environment in which to grow. All these must be provided to result, nine months after conception, in a healthy baby. What you eat and do is also important for you – the parents – to feel physically able to enjoy your new baby, whether it is your first or a sibling. This is how you grow a healthy baby:

a healthy egg and sperm

The basic genetic material which lies at the heart of each newly fertilised egg is the most important factor in determining how the child will develop. The ability to produce eggs and sperm, which are genetically sound, is enhanced by providing the nutritional building blocks for these life-givers.

nourishment to develop

Given that the cells must divide billions of times to result in a baby there is plenty of scope for things to go wrong, and it is miraculous that Mother Nature gets it as right as she normally does! In order for cells to divide properly they need the right raw materials for cell membranes, which are then able to form new 'daughter' cells. All your baby's organs, plus the nervous system, brain, bones, muscles and blood will come from the food you put into your mouth. If you are not able to provide good quality building blocks, the developing foetus may well grow soundly anyway, though possibly not optimally, and at the cost of your own health being compromised.

a safe environment

Cushioned inside your womb for nine months your baby is protected from the outside world. However, sometimes the outside world intrudes and 'womb pollution' can have an effect on the developing foetus. Substances circulating in the mother's blood will, for the most part, be able to cross the placenta and affect the baby. The bald truth is that each time you drink alcohol or coffee, take medication or smoke a cigarette, so does your baby. These substances interfere with the correct use of the building blocks just mentioned because they reduce the uptake of nutrients (vitamins and minerals) and so they are called anti-nutrients. Other pollutants may also be found in the womb environment, including residues from household cleaning materials and farming and industrial chemicals. It is possible to minimise all of these.

WHAT YOU EAT NOW AFFECTS YOUR BABY'S LATER HEALTH

Before your baby can let you know what it wants, he or she must trust you to supply all the nutrients needed for optimal wellbeing. Not only will your diet intimately affect your pregnancy and the immediate development and health of your baby, there is also plenty of evidence that health in childhood and adulthood is also affected by the maternal diet during the pregnancy. There is an increased risk of short attention span problems, hyperactivity, cognitive learning problems, poor concentration, slow reaction to stimuli and slow learning in the children of mothers who were not optimally nourished during pregnancy, and the strain of this on parents, let alone the child, is more than can be put into words.

Your baby inherits a genetic blueprint from you and your partner which determines many traits – from hair colour to temperament. Among that genetic programming may be certain weaknesses – for instance, your family may have a tendency to develop heart disease or diabetes. While you can't change the genes your baby inherits, you can make daily food choices that help limit the development of these family traits. If your baby starts off with an optimally nourished mother, eats well in childhood and develops a lifelong habit of healthy eating and exercise the tendency towards, say, diabetes may never develop.

In adulthood the offspring of mothers who had poor nutrition have a significantly increased risk of problems such as high cholesterol, high blood pressure, poor liver function, heart disease, strokes and diabetes. The whole truth is that it is not just maternal nutrition during pregnancy that counts, but also the 'background' nutrition – the quality of her diet in the years prior to pregnancy, and her nutritional status as she goes into pregnancy.

COUNTDOWN

Many women only start to think about adjusting their diet and lifestyle once they know they are pregnant. At best this can be two weeks after conception, though often it can be two, three or even four months into the pregnancy. The first three months of the pregnancy, however, is the time when the baby is developing from a fertilised egg into a fully formed human being. After that time all the most important organ and nervous tissue developments have taken place and from then on it is mostly a matter of further maturation and growth. It is therefore far better to plan ahead, if you are able, to optimise the environment for your baby in those first few crucial weeks. Outlined here is a six-month countdown to the time when you would like to start trying for a baby. Use these months to look after yourself, to make a safe 'home' for your baby.

SIX MONTHS TO CONCEPTION

- Stop taking the contraceptive pill, and use barrier methods of contraception.
- Make sure both you and your partner are tested for chlamydia and other STDs (see **Check Ups** below). Other check-ups should ideally include testing for toxoplasmosis, German measles, diabetes and thyroid function.
- Stop smoking.
- Start following a wholefood diet (see **Eating for a Perfect Pregnancy**, page 49).
- Start to avoid unnecessary exposure to chemicals in the house and garden, and in foods and drinks (see **The Womb: A Pollution-free Zone**, page 17).

Stop Taking the Pill

It is advisable to stop taking the Pill at least three, and preferably six, months before you plan to conceive, so that your body can return to its natural cycle. At least three normal menstrual cycles should elapse before you try for a baby.

Taking the Pill affects your body in a number of ways. It lowers levels of many nutrients, particularly B-vitamins, including the all-important B-vitamin for pregnancy, folic acid. It also, along with some types of intra-uterine devices (IUDs), raises blood copper levels, which can have the effect of lowering levels of zinc. Zinc is one of the more important nutrients for growth of a baby. Stopping the Pill in plenty of time, and eating zinc-rich foods, allows any deficit to be redressed (see **Eating for a Perfect Pregnancy**, page 76, for sources of zinc). The Pill can also increase the likelihood of developing thrush, as it changes the mucus and bacterial balance in the vagina. As the chances of developing thrush are also compounded by pregnancy, this is another reason to give yourself several Pill-free months before pregnancy.

Natural Family Planning

During the three to six months that you may be preparing for conception you will need to practise family planning methods which do not involve the contraceptive pill or the intra-uterine device (IUD). If you have an IUD fitted it needs to be removed at least one month prior to planned conception. Should you get pregnant while an IUD is in place, speak to your doctor about the pros and cons of leaving it in position throughout the pregnancy or having it removed in the early stages. The most common means of contraception at this time is a barrier method such as the condom or the cap. It may be prudent to avoid spermicides, as you would any other chemical, in the run-up to conception, but if you fall pregnant whilst using them do not worry, as it seems that they are not responsible for increasing the risk of congenital defects. You may also want to use ovulation prediction methods to either avoid making love at fertile times in the few months before you plan conception, or to make love at fertile times if you are hoping to conceive. The three main methods of checking when, and if, you are ovulating include keeping a note of your temperature, checking the viscosity of your cervical mucus or using ovulation predictor kits available from chemists (see **Resources**, page 197).

Check Ups

Now is the time to visit your doctor to check for conditions that are known to affect the chances of having a healthy pregnancy. If any of these are found to be a problem, then your doctor will be able to offer advice and treatment before you get pregnant. These are the main conditions to be concerned about:

german measles
This is the popular name for rubella. If the mother catches this disease during pregnancy, especially in the first three months, it can lead to serious defects in the foetus, including blindness, deafness and heart disease. Your doctor will recommend a blood test pre-conceptually to see if you are immune or if you need to be vaccinated.

toxoplasmosis
This is a protozoa parasite that is found in raw meat and in cat faeces. Toxoplasmosis is also sometimes found in raw goat's and ewe's milk, so you need to ensure that you drink only pasteurised milks. Infection is quite often symptomless, and

around 50 per cent of women are thought to be infected already, meaning that they will have antibodies to toxoplasmosis and their pregnancy will be unaffected. But if a woman, who does not have antibodies, is infected with toxoplasmosis during their pregnancy it can cause serious problems, including birth defects, brain damage and blindness or the foetus may miscarry. Toxoplasmosis affects around two in every thousand pregnancies, or 1,400 babies a year in the UK, and of those ten per cent will have serious damage as a consequence. The test for toxoplasmosis is a standard blood test that is freely available upon request from your doctor.

During, and just before, pregnancy it is important to cook meat thoroughly (see page 102) and to avoid coming into contact with cat faeces. Avoid emptying litter trays, or digging in the garden, without gloves. Even if you do not own a cat, your garden can still be used by those belonging to your neighbours. If you happen to work on a farm, or visit a children's 'petting' farm, make sure that you do not touch lambs or ewes that have recently given birth.

chlamydia

This is a sexually transmitted disease (STD) that is symptomless in 70 per cent of infected women and in 50 per cent of infected men, and is the most common infection transmitted from mother to baby. It is also a common reason for infertility in both women and men. Chlamydia affects one in 14 sexually active people. It can be contracted years previously and lie dormant, only springing to life when you get pregnant. In Sweden, where chlamydia is routinely screened for, the infection rate has halved in the last ten years and there has been a significant decrease in infertility problems. During the same period the rate of chlamydia has increased in the UK. A UK government survey of hundreds of doctors regarding what they believed to be the most dangerous infectious diseases found that chlamydia is rated the third biggest risk to public health, behind HIV and meningitis. In nearly 40 per cent of women with chlamydia it leads to pelvic inflammatory disease (PID), a severe and widespread inflammation of the whole area. If left untreated during pregnancy, it can lead to ectopic pregnancies, miscarriage and eye infections in the baby (sometimes severe). The test is usually a simple swab around the cervix, though more recently a urine test has been developed. Treatment is a course of antibiotics for both partners, as one can re-infect the other.

While no-one likes to think about sexually transmitted diseases, and even if you think you are an unlikely candidate for infection, it is worth asking your doctor for tests. Infections which can be checked for at the same time as chlamydia are gonorrhoea, syphilis, non-specific vaginitis (bacterial vaginitis or Gardnerella vaginitis), genital warts, herpes and HIV. It is also a good idea to be checked for hepatitis B and C. Some of these tests, such as that for syphilis, are routine during antenatal checks, however it is more responsible, and more useful, to be tested pre-conceptually when they can be treated without any harm to the baby.

diabetes

One of the tests that your doctor will routinely run when you are pregnant is a simple urine test to detect the presence of sugar, which may indicate that you are diabetic (though it may just indicate a sugary meal previously). Diabetes is hugely on the increase, a result of the massive increase in sugar, sugary foods and refined carbohydrates in our diet over the last few decades. The average diabetic remains undiagnosed for seven years, and one million people in the UK are currently thought to be undiagnosed diabetics; inevitably a proportion of these will be women in their fertile years aiming for a pregnancy.

If a diabetic woman becomes pregnant, she will be closely monitored, as damage to the kidneys and eyes can be exacerbated by pregnancy.

Pregnancy-related diabetes (gestational diabetes, which can come on during pregnancy) is covered in more detail in **Eating for a Perfect Pregnancy**, page 116.

underfunctioning thyroid
The thyroid hormones are responsible for metabolism, and govern the efficiency of energy production in each and every cell. Because of this, if there is a deficiency of either of the thyroid hormones, there is an increased risk of not being able to maintain the pregnancy, of early miscarriage or of infertility in the first place.

This test is not normally given specifically as a pre-conceptual exercise, however if your doctor thinks that you have symptoms which suggest that low thyroid hormones may be a problem, he or she should be willing to order the test. Symptoms of low thyroid hormone levels include low body temperature, feeling chilly when others feel comfortable, a tendency to put on weight, tiredness not related to lack of sleep, low energy and blood sugar dips or a coarsening of the skin.

Quit Smoking
Giving up smoking is probably the most important thing you can do to promote the health of your baby, and giving up well before you conceive is most useful. A quarter of the 600,000 women who fall pregnant annually in the UK do not give up smoking, which means that a staggering 150,000 babies are born to women who smoke. There are 4,000 harmful chemicals and substances in cigarette smoke, including nicotine, cyanide, nitrosamines, sometimes DDT, and the heavy metals cadmium

and arsenic. These affect the baby directly – carbon monoxide, for example, affects foetal blood flow and the synthesis of brain DNA, nicotine affects foetal heart rate and reduces placental blood flow, polycyclic aromatic hydrocarbons interfere with placental hormones and increase the rate of cell mutations, while cyanide is involved in retarded growth.

If you are having trouble getting pregnant, smoking may be responsible, as it lowers levels of the female hormones oestrogen and progesterone. When pregnant, smoking deprives the baby of oxygen and babies of mothers who smoke are far more likely to be premature or of low birth weight, and have a small head circumference. These can contribute to impaired mental development, a short attention span or hyperactivity in the child. The reason smoking affects birth weight is that it slows down the rate at which the baby grows in the uterus. The cadmium in cigarette smoke is a potent 'anti-nutrient' and competes with the minerals zinc and iron, both of which are vital for a healthy pregnancy. One researcher said, rather chillingly, 'Babies are literally swimming in this carcinogen [cancer-causing substance] and drinking it into their developing bodies.' Smoking (before, during or after pregnancy) also increases the chance of miscarriage, stillbirth and cot death.

It is just as important for both partners to avoid smoking. The father's sperm quality is affected by smoking, and the effects of passive smoking on the mother and the newborn baby can lead to complications. Small children of parents who smoke are more likely to have respiratory problems such as bronchitis and asthma, and compromised immune systems leading to lowered resistance to pneumonia, middle ear infections (glue ear) and meningitis. It is estimated that 17,000 children under the age of five are admitted to hospital each year as a direct result of being affected by passive smoking. It has been identified as one of the main factors involved in the risk of cot death, and 125 babies die each year in the UK as a result of their parents smoking. It has even been established that you do not need to smoke near the child to affect their health. Coming close to them within 30 minutes of smoking a cigarette is sufficient to increase their exposure to damaging chemicals.

While the number of men who smoke is at last decreasing slightly, as women increasingly adopt more male-pattern behaviour the number of female smokers is, unfortunately, rising sharply. Thankfully many women find the resolve to stop when they know they are pregnant, though in an ideal world they would do so pre-conceptually. They also need to maintain their resolve after the birth and and not resume smoking, which is what many women end up doing.

The Womb: A Pollution-Free Zone

There are many sources of chemicals in our environment which can potentially be damaging to a developing baby. These are some of the most obvious to avoid:

- If you, or your partner, has a job that involves working with chemicals, lead, anaesthetics or X-rays these can influence your chances of conception or have an effect on the developing baby. Women are entitled by law to be moved to a job that is not dangerous while they are pregnant.
- Avoid inhaling fumes from cleaning products, paint, lacquers, petrol, aerosols and glue. If you are planning to decorate the baby's new room, use water soluble paints or ask someone else to do the work if possible.
- The average household buys 36 aerosol spray cans per year. A study of 14,000 pregnant women found that those who used the most sprays had 25 per cent more headaches than those who used them least (no mention was made of whether their

babies also got more headaches!). Additionally, they had a 19 per cent greater chance of postnatal depression.

● Avoid using pesticides and chemicals in the garden or house.

● Do not use hair dyes just before and during pregnancy.

● Avoid plastics which can leach harmful hormone-like chemicals in to food and water and which are suspected of contributing to poor sexual maturation in baby boys. Instead of cling-film use baking parchment (secure with a second layer of aluminium if necessary), avoid plastic storage containers, do not cook in plastic packaging and use glass or ceramic, instead of plastic, containers.

● Filter your drinking water (replacing the filter frequently and cleaning the housing to avoid bacteria build-up) or use good quality mineral water (not spring water which is not rigidly regulated), preferably bought in glass bottles.

● Eat organic food whenever you are able to avoid farming chemicals.

● Take a supplement, such as a prenatal formula (see page 20), to help eliminate some of the pollutants to which you are exposed.

● For more information about providing a pollution-free womb see **Nutrient Robbers**, page 71.

THREE MONTHS TO CONCEPTION

● Reduce alcohol intake to a bare minimum, but certainly no more than four measures per week.

● Start taking a vitamin and mineral supplement specially formulated for pregnancy which includes 400 mcg of folic acid (see below).

● If you are not already doing so, work on your stress and fitness levels.

Alcohol

Along with smoking, drinking alcohol is on the increase in women, particularly in the 18–25 year old age group, and this may well result in problems for the next generation. The time when it is most important to avoid alcohol in pregnancy is in the first four or five months when the foetus is most vulnerable to its effects, and yet the first few weeks after conception is the time when a mother is most likely to be drinking because she is unaware she is pregnant. This can cause a lot of worry to women who are acutely aware that they have been drinking as normal and possibly had a few 'heavy sessions' in the first few weeks of their pregnancy. Over indulgence might even have been responsible for conception!

Should they worry? Well, there is no point worrying about something you can't change and, given that babies are quite sturdy little things, the chances are high that everything will be OK. Nevertheless, the evidence is pretty clear that alcohol can be related to a host of problems and it is wise, if possible, to cut back to four units a week a few months before conception, to cut it out completely in the few weeks before conception, and to keep this up for the duration of the pregnancy. One unit is one bar-measure glass of wine, or one measure of spirits or half a pint of normal strength beer.

Some women, because of their metabolism, are unable to fully break down alcohol into less harmless substances. Babies take twice as long to metabolise alcohol, which means that alcohol (which is passed through the placenta to the baby just as quickly as it circulates around your blood) will have twice the effect. When you are feeling tipsy, the baby is getting seriously drunk. So if you are tempted by a drink, remember that you wouldn't put wine in a baby's bottle, so why do it now?

Nobody really knows what the safe limit for alcohol is

during pregnancy, but in the absence of a consensus of opinion the best advice is to take the only really safe approach, and to cut it out altogether. Alcohol acts as an anti-nutrient and depletes B-vitamins in particular (including the all important folic acid which is protective against spina bifida). Even one or two drinks daily is related to an increased risk of miscarriage, stillbirth, developmental problems and growth abnormalities. Alcohol, even in moderation, affects birth weight, and a low birth weight is linked to a variety of problems, including reduced mental development. The baby's nervous system is still developing up until birth, and in fact continues to go through a 'linking-up' process for the first two years afterwards. If you absolutely have to have a drink, a little bit in the last half of the pregnancy, once the baby is mostly formed, is likely to do least harm, but make sure it is accompanied by a meal to slow down its impact on the baby.

As alcohol is the most socially acceptable 'drug', it is a problem for most sectors of society. Foetal alcohol syndrome can be induced by around ten units of alcohol daily, which is about one bottle of wine. The signs of foetal alcohol syndrome, which affects about one or two in a thousand births, are easy to recognise and the most obvious signs are low birth weight and a slightly flattened and misshapen face. Other effects can include heart murmurs, persistent ear infections leading to deafness, fingers and toes that may be malformed and congenital hip dislocation.

Taking Supplements Pre-conceptually

The role of specific nutrients in the development of a healthy baby is covered in detail in **Eating for a Perfect Pregnancy**, page 49. There is no substitute for eating healthily to promote a happy pregnancy, and it is foolish to take a supplement in the belief that this gives leeway for dietary indiscretions. Diet and lifestyle have far more impact on your baby's health than a daily vitamin pill.

However, there is a case for taking supplements pre-conceptually, for the duration of the pregnancy (prenatally) and for the few postnatal months. They can be thought of as 'insurance', to make sure that you and your baby are getting all the vitamins and minerals you both need. There is plenty of evidence that tells us that optimising nutrient intake during pregnancy is beneficial and that supplements can contribute to better outcomes – easier pregnancies and healthier babies.

The most obvious and best known benefit is for women to take folic acid, which dramatically reduces the incidence of neural tube defects, such as spina bifida, where the spinal column fails to develop properly. Advocates of the sensible use of vitamins and mineral supplements have faced opposition from more conservative quarters. Who would have thought that we would finally see the day when women are now routinely encouraged by the health authorities to take folic acid supplements? And yet despite the widespread publicity, a recent study revealed that 39 per cent of women are still unaware of the importance of supplementing this vitamin.

One of the definitions of an essential nutrient, vitamin or mineral, is if fertility and reproductive ability is impaired by its absence. As the diets of most women are in fact deficient in at least one nutrient, it seems obvious to me that along with addressing diet, lifestyle and environmental habits taking a multi-vitamin and mineral supplement is wise in pregnancy. The ideal way to take a supplement is as a multi-nutrient that is designed to give the right balance of vitamins and minerals in relation to each other. As nutrients all work together this is the best way of getting the right levels. For instance, you can certainly take folic acid on its own, but as it works in conjunction with vitamins B12 and B6 it is more effective when taken in combination with these. In addition, taking individual supplements of either folic acid or B12 can mask a deficiency in the other nutrient not being taken. Pregnancy is not the time to experiment with different doses and there are many good quality, well designed, prenatal products (some of which are listed in **Resources**). It is essential to buy reliable products that are formulated with nutrients in their most absorbable form.

Do not be tempted to take a supplement which is not a prenatal formula, as there are some substances which are contra-indicated during pregnancy. Vitamin A in high levels, for example, poses a possible danger to a developing baby and the pregnancy formulas do not use more than around 5,000 ius/1500 mcg (μg) daily. In addition, they are mostly based on beta-carotene, which converts into vitamin A as needed, with the excess excreted harmlessly. Apart from taking a multi-supplement containing lower amounts of vitamin A, you also need to pick an antioxidant formula that uses beta-carotene (they usually include vitamin A – also called retinol or palmitol). Another source of high doses of vitamin A from supplements is cod liver oil. If you have been taking any of this whilst unaware that you are pregnant do not worry, recent studies suggest that the sort of levels that this would expose a baby to in the first few weeks would probably not do any harm, just switch as soon as possible. The current wisdom is that it is best to avoid the compound effect of taking a multi-supplement with vitamin A alongside an antioxidant with vitamin A and also a cod liver oil supplement (a combination which is not uncommon).

Another reason for taking a prenatal formula, instead of a 'normal' formula is that the special formulas do not use herbs which need to be avoided in pregnancy. If you are taking any herbal supplements, including energy boosters such as ginseng or liquorice root, stop immediately and consult a professional herbalist for advice about the safe use of herbs during pregnancy. The chapter **The Natural Remedy Cupboard** takes you through the use of some herbs which can be useful in pregnancy.

what to look for in a daily pregnancy-formulated supplement programme

what	why
folic acid – 400 mcg, preferably combined with 25 mcg B12 and 25 mg each of the other B-vitamins	protects against the risk of spina bifida
zinc – 15 mg	used for all growth processes
vitamin E – 400 ius/270 mg as d-alpha tocopherol	an antioxidant which may help to protect against pre-eclampsia
vitamin C – 1,000 mg (1 g)	for collagen formation and an antioxidant (see above)
calcium – 250 mg, and **magnesium** – 150 mg	for bone health and to help protect against pre-eclampsia
iron – 10 mg of elemental iron	for blood formation
vitamin D – 200 ius/5 mcg	to support bone health
vitamin A – 5,000 ius/1,500 mcg (µg) maximum	or use a product with an equivalent amount of beta-carotene
chromium – 50–100 mcg	to help reduce the risk of blood sugar problems
selenium – 50 mcg	antioxidant mineral
flax oil – 1 gm capsule	for essential fats

This is an ideal programme for most women in reasonable health. You will not get all of the above in one supplement, and you will need to take a separate multi-vitamin and multi-mineral tablet, along with a gram of vitamin C and a gram of flax oil.

Stress

A relaxed parent is the most essential ingredient for a relaxed child. Perhaps now is the time to get serious about doing relaxation exercises, taking time out for yourself and addressing any pressing issues that need to be resolved. The effects of stress on the body are significant and can contribute to high blood pressure, tense muscles, inefficient digestion, depression and many other symptoms. Ultrasound scans have shown that anxiety in pregnancy can lead to a reduced blood flow to the baby and high levels of stress may increase the risk of pre-term babies. In the most anxious mothers the blood flow was so badly impaired that it became of clinical significance.

It also seems that couples who find it harder to conceive may be affected by their stress levels. Conception rates are much higher during holidays when, it is presumed, people are more relaxed and under less stress. It could also be that they have more energy for sex, being too tired normally, in which case there is even more reason to pay attention to nutritional status. One study also showed that women who enjoy sex have more live sperm afterwards in their cervical mucus than women who do not get much pleasure from it.

Learning to pace yourself during your pregnancy is no bad thing, and your hormone changes, with rising levels of proges-terone, are likely to incline you to take life at a slower pace, so don't fight it too much!

Exercise

Staying fit and flexible is a great boon, helping to ensure a healthy pregnancy. If you are planning to get pregnant in the next few months you can also optimise your health by starting, or continuing, an exercise programme. There is no reason why most women should not continue to exercise throughout their pregnancy, as long as they also 'exercise' some common sense, and check with their doctor or midwife first. For women who are following a regular fitness programme before pregnancy, limit your heart rate to a maximum of 140 beats per minute during pregnancy to ensure that you are not exercising at too high an intensity. It is better to exercise regularly, three or four times a week, rather than to skip sessions and then try to 'catch-up'. Make sure, too, that you always warm-up and cool-down from your exercise programme, and that you drink plenty of water before, during and after your work-out session so that you and your baby stay hydrated, and to counter a raised body temperature.

Exercise increases your sense of well-being and is a great idea for optimising your pregnancy. Mothers who burn 1,000 calories a week during exercise have babies, on average, five per cent heavier than the norm, and heavier babies are healthier and have better developed immune systems than smaller babies.

benefits of exercise before and during pregnancy include

- relieves backache
- prevents constipation
- reduces risk of varicose veins
- fewer pregnancy complications
- fewer obstetric interventions
- less pregnancy-related diabetes
- an easier labour
- lower risk of pre-eclampsia

contraindications for exercise during pregnancy include

- previous miscarriages
- previous pre-term labour
- previous ruptured membranes
- pregnancy induced high blood
  pressure
- incompetent cervix
- history of bleeding in pregnancy
- multiple foetuses
- cardiovascular or pulmonary
  disease, or asthma

If you have not already embarked on an exercise regime, pregnancy is the wrong time to start a vigorous campaign. However, you can certainly begin a more gentle movement regime. Many women find that yoga is invaluable in pregnancy, helping them to relax and meditate as well as allowing them to limber up, stretch muscles and strengthen the back in preparation for the main event. Always tell the yoga teacher if you are pregnant as some moves may not be advised, or positions may not be held for quite such a long time, but generally yoga is a discipline that relies on slow, smooth movements and correctly held postures that can easily be carried out in pregnancy.

Keeping fit during pregnancy will help to control an excess increase in body weight, and can act to calm the emotions. Apart from yoga, ideal exercise options during pregnancy for the not very fit include walking briskly and swimming (where your body weight is supported and your back can be strengthened). Even if you don't follow a specific exercise routine, take time out for a daily half-hour walk, and learn to put your feet up for a further half an hour a day.

ONE MONTH TO CONCEPTION

● Avoid all alcohol.
● Have your IUD (intra-uterine device) removed and
  stop using spermicides. Use barrier methods without
  spermicides until you are ready to try for a baby.

- Avoid over-the-counter drugs. Speak to your doctor about the effects of any prescription medication you are taking.
- Moderate or cut out caffeine.
- Continue to eat a wholefood diet as outlined in **Eating for a Perfect Pregnancy**, page 49, and take your pregnancy-formulated vitamins and minerals up to and throughout your pregnancy.

Drugs and Medicines

Some drugs and medicines can affect fertility or be damaging to the developing baby. Avoid all over-the-counter and recreational drugs, and speak to your doctor about the likely effects of any prescribed medication you are taking upon the health of your baby. If you are consulting a doctor, pharmacist, herbalist, nutritionist or other health practitioner always mention that you are planning to conceive, or that you are pregnant.

If you have a problem with giving up any recreational drugs, or alcohol, speak to a counsellor as soon as you can. Frankly, you need to consider postponing pregnancy until you are sure you can stay clean. The use of drugs before pregnancy is unlikely to be a major problem in terms of direct toxicity effects on the baby, though they will probably have acted as anti-nutrients, which means that you need to be more assiduous about your diet (see **Nutrient Robbers**, page 71). You must make sure that you can stay off drugs during pregnancy, including seemingly benign drugs such as marijuana. Even infrequent use of drugs such as marijuana and cocaine are linked to hazards such as low-birth weight babies, foetal alcohol syndrome-like characteristics and behavioural problems. Many types of drugs can also lead to congenital defects in the baby.

Medicine	Possible effect on the baby
amphetamines	heart defects
antihistamines	malformations
anti-nausea	malformations
aspirin	prevents blood clotting
codeine	addictive
diuretics	blood disorders
paracetamol	liver damage
phenytoin (epilepsy)	malformations
steroids	hormonal
streptomycin (antibiotic)	deafness
sulphonamides (antibiotics)	birth jaundice
tetracycline (antibiotic)	yellow teeth
Valium	respiratory problems

This chart does not cover all drugs, but only some of the most common. If a drug is not mentioned this does not imply that it is safe. Check with your doctor.

Caffeine
. . . .

Caffeine is a drug. There is no mistaking this when you find yourself getting headaches, feeling sluggish and craving your fix, as many people do when they try to give it up. It is a stimulant which will cross the placental barrier and hype up the baby just as much as yourself. During pregnancy caffeine is broken down in the liver three times more slowly than normally, so it can have an even greater effect on your sleeping patterns, as well as the baby's ability to rest and sleep in the womb. Some studies show that the time to conception is longer in those who drink around 500 mg of caffeine. Other studies associate three cups of coffee (250–300 mg caffeine) with an increased risk of miscarriage. It is generally advised, however, that 300 mg of caffeine a day is safe, in that it does not seem to result in congenital problems for the baby. How fair is it, however, to impose such a strong stimulant on your baby (remember the jolt when you had your first coffee)?

The other problem with caffeinated drinks such as coffee and tea, is that they limit the absorption of nutrients, particularly zinc and B-vitamins from food, so a post-prandial coffee will actually reduce the overall nutritional benefit of a meal by around 25 per cent. Caffeine also encourages the excretion of calcium. It is probably best to limit yourself while pregnant to two or three weak teas, avoid coffee and enjoy some of the excellent substitutes that are widely available. Experiment with chicory, dandelion and barley coffees, as well as fruit teas, but be cautious about herbal teas (see **The Natural Remedy Cupboard**, page 119). You can also use decaffeinated versions of teas and coffee, though it is best to choose naturally decaffeinated brands (this will be mentioned on the labels) which avoid solvents.

caffeine contents (averages)

	serving	*caffeine (mg)*
ground coffee	1 150-ml cup	60–150mg
espresso/cappuccino	single shot	50 mg
instant coffee	1 150-ml cup	30–90 mg
tea – strong	1 150-ml cup	50 mg
tea – weak	1 150-ml cup	30 mg
decaf coffee/tea	1 150 ml cup	2–4 mg
cola	1 can	30–40 mg
dark (bitter) chocolate	100 g	40–70 mg
milk chocolate	100 g	5–30 mg

AVOIDING INFECTIONS DURING PREGNANCY

There are diseases that you need to avoid if you are pregnant as they can affect the developing foetus. These include German measles (if you are not immune), chickenpox, fifth disease, hand-foot-and-mouth disease and cytomegalovirus. If you are around children, or adults, who develop fever, rashes or any other symptoms it is wise to avoid contact with them until they have had a correct diagnosis from a doctor. In the meantime, ask non-pregnant friends or relatives to nurse any sick children you have. Likewise, avoid anyone with colds and coughs and stomach bugs, and this goes for strangers on the bus who may splutter all over you just as much as your nearest and dearest.

FERTILITY

When an egg is released it is only viable for one day, after which it degenerates and cannot be fertilised. Sperm, on the other hand, can remain viable in the environment of the cervix, womb and fallopian tubes for up to four days, sometimes longer. To optimise the chances of getting pregnant it is best to be aware of when you ovulate, and to make love with your partner as much as possible during the two or three days before ovulation and on the days of and following ovulation. Of course, premeditated love-making such as this can be a real turn-off for some couples, and there is a strong case for relaxing and letting nature take its course. It is not unheard of for couples who have been living by charts for many months, to succeed once they threw them away!

If you find that you do not conceive within a time span that you think is reasonable, your doctor can run tests to determine whether you are ovulating successfully and whether you are maintaining the right hormone levels after ovulation to maintain a pregnancy. If the woman is under the age of 35 it is generally considered that up to a year is a reasonable time period to wait for conception before making other investigations. If she is over 35, six months is the time span usually allowed to elapse before investigations are made.

One in five couples find that they have trouble conceiving. However, in many cases infertility may actually be *sub*-fertility, and the chances of successful conception increase in relation to the attention paid to nutritional status, and avoiding smoking, alcohol and anxiety.

reasons for infertility can include

woman
- blocked fallopian tubes
- endometriosis
- pelvic inflammatory disease
- polycystic ovaries
- poor quality eggs (ova)
- being seriously underweight or overweight
- low thyroid function
- insufficient progesterone hormone produced to maintain a pregnancy
- antiphospholipid disorder (the cause of 1 in 6 recurrent miscarriages), where maternal antibodies increase the risk of blood clotting; often treated with low dose aspirin and heparin, which increases the pregnancy success rate from 10 per cent to 75 per cent. Vitamin E (400-800 ius) and fish oils also thin blood but this condition must always be discussed with your doctor

man
- low sperm count
- poor sperm motility
- poor quality sperm

both partners
- alcohol, cigarette or drug use

● poor nutritional status
● infections, such as chlamydia

One intriguing study conducted by Foresight (see **Resources**) and Surrey University looked at 418 couples, three quarters of whom had a history of previous infertility or miscarriage. They had their diets analysed for deficiencies and for vitamin, mineral and toxic heavy metal levels (see **Nutrient Robbers**, page 71). All alcohol, sugar and refined and processed foods were eliminated from their diets, along with any foods to which they were thought to be sensitive (dairy produce and gluten grains such as wheat). This experiment proved to be highly successful, with 81 per cent of the couples conceiving and having healthy babies. There were no miscarriages, perinatal deaths or deformities, no babies needed to go to the special care unit, none were born before 36 weeks and none were lighter than 2.35 kg/5 lb 3 oz.

If you have had problems with fertility you may need to pay attention to nutrient levels, in particular levels of vitamin E, magnesium, zinc, selenium and essential fats. Low levels of selenium (found in nuts, seafood, wholegrains and pulses), for example, have been observed in women who miscarry, and it is likely that low selenium levels are linked to an increase in DNA damage. High levels of toxic heavy metals, such as lead and cadmium, may inhibit pregnancy.

The implications of exposure to environmental chemical hazards is probably going to be recognised as a time-bomb for fertility. The average tissue sample today from an adult contains 400-500 synthetic chemicals, whereas samples taken from Egyptian mummies contain virtually none. The effects of most chemicals on fertility can only be guessed at at the moment, but if you are having trouble conceiving then take this matter seriously. Low level toluene exposure experienced by women in the printing industry, for example, is linked to lowered fertility, and female textile workers have also been discovered to have high levels of the chemicals found in carpets, wood preservative treatments and upholstery. So, as well as following the advice given in **Eating for a Perfect Pregnancy**, page 49, clean up your environment by banishing unnecessary chemicals.

PREVIOUS MISCARRIAGES

Miscarriage is defined as losing a pregnancy before 24 weeks. It is estimated that one in four pregnancies ends in miscarriage in the first three months, often without the mother ever being aware of what has happened. She may experience nothing more troubling than an unusually heavy period or a haemorrhaging at a time when her period is not normally due, but which may be mistaken for an early period. It is also estimated that the majority of early miscarriages come about because of an abnormality in the embryo due to genetic irregularities or infection, and over half studied have had chromosomal defects. Two in five miscarriages, however, remain unexplained.

The main aim of this chapter is to ensure that the conditions are optimal to prevent this happening. If you have previously experienced a miscarriage, it becomes even more important to observe the pre-conceptual planning period, and it is best to wait for three months before trying for a baby again. If you have miscarried before, however, the good news is that the risk of a second miscarriage is relatively low compared to the first time round, and only 1 per cent of women are affected by recurrent miscarriages. Of course, a woman who miscarries may well be grieving quite profoundly (something that is not always acknowledged by the woman herself or the people around her). If this is the case, the motivation to look after herself, and to cook and eat healthily, can be blunted. Nevertheless, it is wise to think about all aspects of your own health and that of your partner. You may need to look in less than obvious places for clues. For instance, one study showed that women who used VDUs for more than 20 hours a week were twice as likely to have a miscarriage as those who did not use VDUs.

If you have a history of repeat miscarriages seek out a nutritionally trained doctor or a nutritionist specialising in pre-conceptual care to assess your nutritional status. Your status for all nutrients will need to be checked, in particular levels of zinc, red cell magnesium, copper and essential fats, as well as toxic metals such as lead and cadmium. Raised levels of a toxic substance called homocysteine, which around 25 per cent of people are prone to have if they do not get sufficient folic acid or vitamins B12 or B6, is linked to recurrent spontaneous mis-carriages, as well as to abruptio placenta (bleeding or detached placenta after about 24 weeks). In a study of 130 women, only 9 per cent of women with normal pregnancies had elevated homocysteine while 31 per cent of women with abruptio placenta had raised levels. Co-enzyme Q10, an antioxidant, may also be a factor – a study of 500 pregnant women showed that CoQ10 levels naturally rise with each trimester but low levels were noted in those with spontaneous abortions.

MATURE PREGNANCIES

A growing number of women (and this included me) are having babies after the age of 35, or even later in their 40s, and there does not seem to be any slowing down of this trend. This choice has advantages and disadvantages. The most likely complication is that, after waiting this long, a woman may find it more difficult to conceive. Beyond the age of 30 a woman is likely to have fewer cycles during which she ovulates, and as she ages the viability of her eggs is likely to decrease. A 35-year-old woman takes twice as long, on average, to conceive as does a 25-year-old.

There is also a slight increase in the risk of having a Down's syndrome baby, the result of a chromosomal abnormality. This is thought to occur because the quality of the egg's genetic material has deteriorated, either through age, or through a lifetime exposure to X-rays, drugs, infections, chemicals and so on. This chromosomal problem is also linked to defective sperm in 25 per cent of cases. There are tests available to determine the likelihood of the baby you are carrying being affected by Down's syndrome, though some tests carry risks in their own right and the decision making process, if the chances of carrying a Down's baby seem high, may be very difficult for some couples.

Whether the considerations are at the more serious end of the scale (fertility and Down's) or a matter of maintaining energy levels to cope with a lively baby and toddler, the effects of nutrition are fundamental for the 35+ age group. Taking the one factor of advanced reproductive age in isolation is not sufficient to determine that someone is in a high-risk category for these problems. Certainly older mothers are more likely to have built up health problems, with work and stress taking their toll, and an unhealthy lifestyle may have led to vitamin and mineral deficiencies. However, when attention is paid to diet, exercise and lifestyle factors such as smoking and exposure to chemicals, it can sufficiently improve the older woman's risk-factors so that her chances of having a healthy pregnancy and baby equal that of a younger woman. It can also mean she has a similar level of physical stamina to deal with parenting.

BIRTH WEIGHT OF THE BABY

One of the terms that you will see constantly referred to throughout the book is 'low birth weight baby'. A low birth weight baby is technically one which is born weighing less than 2.5 kg (5 lb 8 oz), and 7 per cent of babies fall into this category. Within this category are two types of babies: pre-term, or premature, babies, or small-for-date babies who are born at the right time but do not flourish in the uterus.

Of course, genetically, there will be smaller babies, just as there will be larger babies, and multiple births will also usually produce smaller than average babies. However, the most important factors affecting the weight of a baby are the mother's nutritional status, and her use of cigarettes, alcohol and drugs. The reason that so much attention is paid low birth weight is that it carries with it a higher risk of the baby being stillborn, dying within one month, or suffering from mental handicap, blindness, deafness, epilepsy or autism.

At the other end of the scale, women with diabetes tend to have overly large babies, weighing more than 4.3 kg/9 lb 8 oz. With oversize babies there is an increased risk of upper respiratory tract infections, and early research is also suggests that they may be more prone to asthma. Again the point about this is that adult onset diabetes and gestational diabetes are problems that can mostly be addressed by diet.

SPACING BETWEEN PREGNANCIES

It makes sense that a woman needs to recover her nutrient status after having a baby before embarking on the next pregnancy. Growing another person for nine months, and then feeding and caring for that little person afterwards, can be quite a drain on physical resources. Research backs up the suspicion that a mother needs to recuperate, and the optimal time for conceiving the second baby seems to be 18–24 months after having the first baby (which would mean that the second baby comes along when the first is two and a quarter to three years old). If babies are conceived earlier than this, there is an increased risk of them having a low birth weight or being pre-term, as there just isn't enough nourishment to go round. To a degree, nature takes care of this possibility and less than 50 per cent of breast-feeding women ovulate earlier than six months after their first pregnancy. It takes three months to one year to replenish iron and zinc stores after a pregnancy, and vitamin A and essential fats are also depleted by pregnancy. If you do find yourself pregnant within a short time of your previous baby – either by accident or by design – you have even more reason to stick to Eating for a Perfect Pregnancy and to take a prenatal supplement.

CHAPTER TWO

Man Talk

It takes two to tango, and two to make babies. Whilst, in the past, books about pregnancy were aimed solely at the woman, no self-respecting book these days is without a chapter, as well as many references throughout the text, on the role the man plays in supporting his partner through the pregnancy. Men are now viewed as having an essential part to play after conception – through the pregnancy, at antenatal classes, at the birth (all those huffing and puffing fathers) and during child rearing. One of the effects of this is the occasional word of criticism from women who, either through design or circumstance, have a baby on their own, as this can leave them feeling marginalised, and no doubt future books will take into account this rising trend. As this book is about nutrition and pregnancy I do not need to delve into these issues, however what I do need to talk about is the question of how male health affects fertility. Sound eating habits help to provide first rate genetic material for the offspring – sometimes a good sperm can be hard to find!

SPERM QUALITY

It is just as important for a man to prepare for making babies as it is for a woman. After all, his sperm is 50 per cent of the equation in creating a healthy baby. It takes around three months to make a sperm before it is ready for ejaculation, so ensuring a healthy diet and lifestyle for at least four months beforehand is very important. Defective sperm is equally likely to be responsible for birth defects resulting from genetic abnormalities, as is the genetic material from the mother.

Men have experienced an astounding drop in sperm counts in only the last 50 years. Average levels have halved from 113 million sperm per ml to 66 million sperm per ml. When levels drop to 20 million sperm per ml this is classified as a reason for infertility.

It is not just sperm quantity and quality that is a concern. Sperm motility is also critical. Motility means the speed and efficiency with which the sperm swim towards their ultimate destination. As there is a crucial 24 hours in which the egg can be fertilised, they need to be able to move pretty quickly to get up to the fallopian tubes in time for the big meeting. If the sperm are lethargic and lack the 'will' to swim it can make getting pregnant quite difficult.

Most of the advice given for the woman's benefit in **Preparing for a Perfect Pregnancy** and in **Eating for a Perfect Pregnancy** is appropriate for the man in the few months leading up to anticipated conception, and this includes dietary recommendations and testing for STDs such as chlamydia. As for a woman, it is not a good idea for a man to be on a weight-reducing/calorie-restricted diet or an off-the-wall sports diet while trying for a baby, as the reduced nutritional status of such regimes has been shown to reduce sperm formation.

Both smoking and alcohol have been shown to have a detrimental effect on sperm quality and motility. They also have an effect on hormones, and smoking lowers testosterone levels, while alcohol increases female hormones in men (extreme examples are beer-drinking men with breasts). Smoking also lowers seminal vitamin E and other antioxidant levels. Antioxidants are essential for maintaining the genetic integrity of sperm and reducing the risk of mutations. Smoking by the father in the year before conception may well increase the risk of the baby developing leukaemia and certain other cancers – a burden no-one would want to bear. Coffee intake may also be a factor and there is some evidence of spontaneous abortion, premature birth and stillbirth occurring where there is high paternal coffee consumption.

Over-the-counter and recreational drugs need to be avoided as they can also affect sperm production, as can some prescribed drugs, so if you are taking the latter you need to speak to your doctor. Also of great concern is the exposure that some men have in the workplace to chemicals that can affect the genetic material of their sperm, in particular men who work in agriculture and are exposed to farming chemicals. Regular exposure to industrial chemicals or radiation may also result in lower sperm count and possible genetic defects in children.

It is suspected that the main reason why sperm levels have dropped so dramatically in men in the last 50 years is exposure to a wide variety of chemicals in our environment, and in food and water, which mimic the female hormone oestrogen. These chemicals, or xenoestrogens, have been nicknamed 'gender-benders' and they are considerably more potent than the natural hormones women produce in their bodies. (Men also produce some oestrogens but at a much lower level than women.) As well as being linked to female hormonal problems, xenoestrogens are also linked to male hormone and reproductive problems, including low fertility, hypospadias in baby boys (a malformed penis), benign prostate hypertrophy (BHP) and testicular and prostate cancers. Danish research recently showed that sperm counts of men who belonged to their Organic Farmers Association were twice those of ordinary greenhouse workers exposed to herbicides and pesticides. The main sources of xenoestrogens are likely to be plastics, such as cling film and packaging that comes into contact with food and drink, contaminated water, pesticides found on non-organic foods (particularly fatty foods) and dioxins.

There is also some merit in the old-fashioned suggestion that men who want to father a baby need to wear loose underwear. Body temperature is too hot to produce healthy sperm and the testicles are very sensitive to heat. In hot weather they drop, and when it is cold they contract to get closer to body warmth. If you wear tight underwear or trousers all the time then you do not give them the chance to react normally.

NUTRIENTS FOR MALE FERTILITY

A man produces between 100–1,000 million sperm each day (at 100 million that is 1,000 sperm each second) and he needs a healthy diet with maximum nutrient levels to ensure that the majority of these sperm are healthy. In addition to eating a whole-food diet, there are some nutrients which are particularly important for producing healthy sperm.

zinc This is probably the most studied mineral in terms of male fertility and it is vital for male sexual reproductive health. Zinc is needed to make the outer layer and tail of sperm. Long-term deficiencies have been linked to late male sexual development, small genitalia, damaged testes and infertility. Correcting zinc deficiencies can improve or correct some of these conditions, particularly infertility. With 31 per cent of men having insuffi-cient dietary intake, according to Government figures, this means that one in three men who are seeking to father a child may be adversely affected. In addition, men who are very sexually active may well be depleting themselves of this vital mineral as 2–3 mg of zinc are lost in the semen with each ejac-ulation. Zinc is also needed to mobilise vitamin A from liver stores, and vitamin A is needed to make the male sex hormones.

One of the richest sources of zinc is the oyster, which may well be why, throughout history, it has been thought of as a food with aphrodisiac qualities. If your tastes don't quite run to slipping down a few oysters each week (they contain a whopping 80 mg per dozen), other zinc-rich foods include moderate portions of red meat and dark chicken or turkey meat, fresh nuts, pumpkin, sunflower and sesame seeds, and eggs.

If you want to take a zinc supplement, take between 15–25 mg a day. It works best if taken alongside a B-complex that gives at least 50 mg of vitamin B6. If you take this level of zinc for more than three months make sure that the supplement you take includes 1 mg of copper per 10 mg of zinc.

vitamin C Studies suggest that there is an increase in birth defects and childhood illnesses in the offspring of men with low dietary vitamin C. This vitamin plays a crucial role in maintaining levels of sperm counts and sperm motility, and also reduces the clumping of sperm often seen in infertility.

While vitamin C is necessary for everyone (it is used in the metabolism of all cells and is an important antioxidant), it is vital that any potential father who smokes gets more than the recommended amount. Smoking destroys vitamin C at the rate of 25 mg per cigarette, and this may make the link between smoking, low vitamin C and birth defects even more acute. Of course, the best solution is to quit smoking!

Fruit and vegetables, but particularly citrus fruit, strawberries, blackcurrants, kiwis, cabbage and broccoli, are all vitamin C rich foods. If you want to supplement vitamin C, 250–500 mg daily is the lowest meaningful dose, and up to 3 g daily is perfectly safe (for further information, see page 80).

vitamin E A fat-soluble antioxidant that is essential to protect the fatty acids in sperm membranes from oxidation damage.

Sources of vitamin E are cold-pressed oils, fresh nuts and seeds. If you are supplementing vitamin E you need to take between 400–800 ius in its d-alpha-tocopherol form (not dl-alpha-tocopherol). Do not take it, however, alongside blood-thinning medication such as Warfarin without professional advice.

essential fats These are fats that cannot be made in the body and have to be acquired from the diet. They are vital for producing healthy sperm, and the prostaglandins, which are hormone-like substances found in seminal fluid. Highly unsaturated fats, such as these, give flexibility to the cell membranes that make up the sperm. A fat called DHA (decosahexanoic acid), found in fish, is also found in high levels in the testes and is used to make prostaglandins. Supplementing DHA does not dramatically affect these levels, though eating oily fish may help. (For sources of essential fats, see page 54.)

other nutrients A deficiency of magnesium has been linked to chromosomal abnormalities, though this finding has probably also been indicative of a generally low nutritional status. Since magnesium is widely deficient in the diet (42 per cent of men do not get enough, which means two out of every five men hoping to father a child may be affected), it would be wise to eat more magnesium-rich foods, such as nuts and seeds (again!) and dark green leafy vegetables.

Another mineral linked to low sperm count is selenium, which is around 50 per cent deficient in the average diet. It is not as easy to get enough selenium in the diet as it once was, however, as our imported grains now come from selenium deficient areas. One of the simplest ways to get your quota is to eat just three or four Brazil nuts daily.

Another antioxidant, Co-enzyme Q10, or CoQ10 for short, has been shown to enhance sperm motility. CoQ10 is made in the body, but if a person's liver is below par there is a chance that below-optimal amounts are being made. Supplements are available, and around 100 mg daily is likely to be the most effective dose. It is a fat-soluble nutrient, which means that any supplement should include some oil in the capsule.

The B-vitamins, particularly B12 and folic acid, are also important for sperm production. Other nutrients which may help if sperm motility and quality are a problem are three amino acids (protein building blocks) called L-arginine, L-carnitine and L-taurine. If you have a sperm test that highlights problems then supplementing with these amino acids may help, though it is best to get professional nutritional advice before doing so as there are some contra-indications.

A MAN'S ROLE

At the beginning of this chapter I said I would focus on the man's nutritional preparations for fatherhood. There are, of course, other things that the man can do to support his partner and help her to stick to Eating for a Perfect Pregnancy:

- Moral support is always welcome.
- Support your partner's healthy eating choices by eating the same way and encouraging the rest of the family to do so as well.
- Avoid stocking up the larder with convenience foods that your partner might prefer to avoid.
- Bring home extra-delicious treats that support her health programme (mangoes, macadamia nuts or a fragrant Thai curry take-away with brown rice would be some of my choices).
- Be aware of how you can reduce exposure to potentially

toxic chemicals in your household and garden – and do something about it.

● Cook nutritious meals. Help with household chores. Do the weekly shop and come back with foods she is choosing to eat. Help out with the kids.

● Help your partner to build her strength up after one pregnancy and prepare for another.

I am sure that you can think of many other ways to nurture your partner that show you are in tune with her needs.

Part Two

EATING FOR

A PERFECT

PREGNANCY

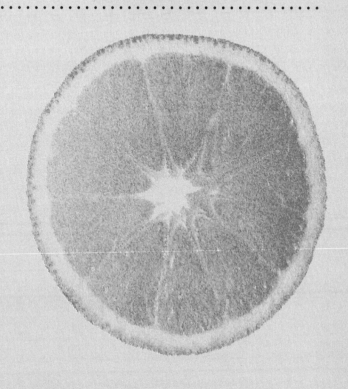

CHAPTER THREE

Eating for a Perfect Pregnancy

Probably the easiest way of ensuring that what you eat benefits you and your baby is to get into the habit of always looking at what you are about to put into your mouth and asking the question 'Is this food going to nourish me and my baby or is this going to detract from our nourishment?' The number one rule of Eating for a Perfect Pregnancy is to make every mouthful count. You may be getting more than enough calories, but they may not be delivering the necessary nutrients.

The 150 calories provided by half a bar of chocolate are in no way equal to the 150 calories provided by a low-fat yoghurt and piece of fruit; the same is true of the nutrients contained in a slice of white toast versus the wholemeal version. Not only does a cup of coffee act as an anti-nutrient (reducing the number of nutrients you absorb from a meal), it also means that the opportunity to drink a hydrating glass of water or a nourishing fruit juice has been lost. Why eat a handful of potato crisps, which are high in hydrogenated fats and salt, when you could be eating fresh nuts or seeds, which will give you calcium, magnesium, vitamin E, zinc, selenium and essential fats? During pregnancy remember that a developing baby has only one source of food – YOU.

Despite popular belief, the need for calories does not increase all that much during pregnancy, although the need for some nutrients can increase by between 30–100 per cent. This means that you need to make sure that the food you eat is *nutrient dense.* More protein, calcium, magnesium and phosphorus are needed for cells which are rapidly dividing, and to form new bones. More iron and B vitamins are needed for your blood supply, which will expand by 35–50 per cent, and for the baby's blood supply. Your need for folic acid doubles as millions of new cells divide to make a new being.

Eating a varied and well balanced diet does not need to be complicated. All it entails is eating foods that are fresh, unprocessed and generally low in sugar and salt. Practically speaking, this means eating as many vegetables, fruits, whole grains, pulses, beans and fish as possible, plus moderate amounts of dairy food, meat and added fats. Keep convenience foods, such as pies, biscuits, crisps, cakes, buns and confectionery (which are mostly low in nutrients, and can even rob you of nutrients) to a bare minimum. You only need an extra 200 calories in your last trimester, so the old adage 'eating for two' clearly does not apply. Two hundred calories is only three extra pieces of fruit, or two slices of bread, or an apple and a yoghurt, or a glass of skimmed milk and a banana.

If you are now thinking 'great advice, but I've never managed to stick to a healthy eating plan before, so how can I manage it now?' don't despair. Your particular concerns are covered later in **Junk Food Junkies**, page 112. For now, read on and learn what is best for your baby and you, and we will work on changing habits later.

THE FOOD PYRAMID

The food pyramid, which is outlined opposite, is the best way of working out if you are achieving a healthy balance of foods in your diet. The foods at the base of the pyramid should be eaten in the greatest amounts.

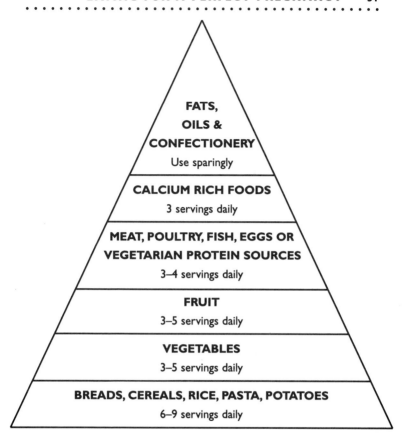

FATS,
OILS &
CONFECTIONERY
Use sparingly

CALCIUM RICH FOODS
3 servings daily

MEAT, POULTRY, FISH, EGGS OR
VEGETARIAN PROTEIN SOURCES
3–4 servings daily

FRUIT
3–5 servings daily

VEGETABLES
3–5 servings daily

BREADS, CEREALS, RICE, PASTA, POTATOES
6–9 servings daily

Fats, Oils, Confectionery

This section concerns *added* fats, such as butter on bread, oils used for dressing salads and for cooking, and any confectionery, whether it is chocolate, snack bars or crisps. These appear at the top of the pyramid because they need to be consumed in the smallest quantities. Generally speaking, they should not add up to more than 15 per cent of your daily total of calories. You obtain sufficient fats from other foods in your diet, such as dairy produce, oily fish, meat, eggs, avocados, nuts and seeds, which easily take you to the recommended amount of fat of 30 per cent of calories. So if you are currently in the first two trimesters of your pregnancy, and are of average build, you need around 2,000 calories daily, of which ideally around 400 calories will be derived from *added* fats, oils and confectionery – that is one level tablespoon of butter, plus one tablespoon of oil, and one-third of a chocolate bar each day. If you are in your third trimester, and need around 2,200 calories daily, this means only another 40 calories from fats, oils and confectionery – which is equivalent to about five potato crisps that you might absentmindedly take from a bowl (whereas you could, instead, have a more satisfying half a baked potato dressed with yoghurt and chives).

Of greater importance than quantity, is the quality of the fats you eat. Margarines made from hydrogenated fats, oils that are not cold-pressed, and meat dripping are the least helpful, and in some instances can be harmful either because they increase oxidation damage or because overuse leads to excess levels of saturated fats. Hydrogenated fats have no useful function in your body, or your baby's, and they contravene the number one rule of Eating for a Perfect Pregnancy – they do not contribute anything useful. The fats that are healthiest for you and your baby are those that are used for building cell membranes, making hormones and for nervous tissue and brain functioning. These are found naturally in foods such as fish, nuts and seeds, but in terms of added oils and fats the healthiest to use are extra-virgin olive oil and cold-pressed flax, walnut, sunflower, safflower and sesame oils.

There is nothing wrong with using a little butter to cook with or to put on your bread, but it is far more beneficial to cook with olive oil and to use other spreads on your bread – though not, however, commercially available low-fat spreads, as these usually just have water whipped into them. While butter merely provides 100 per cent fat, other spreads such as hummus, bean dips and tapenada provide fibre, minerals, essential fats and a better range of vitamins – Eating for a Perfect Pregnancy again. Other spreads to experiment with include almond nut butter, reduced fat cream cheese, home-made mackerel paté (blend smoked mackerel with cottage cheese) and pasteurised mushroom paté.

To keep your use of added fats to a reasonable level learn to cook using low fat methods – stir-fry in a small amount of olive or sesame oil, steam-fry, grill, dry bake (or bake using water and the minimum of oil) or steam, instead of frying, adding a lot of oil to your baking or boiling away nutrients in water. You can always add a teaspoonful or two of an oil such as walnut, sesame or flax to your finished dish to add flavour instead of drenching it in oil whilst cooking.

essential fats

There are some fats that are vital for human health and they are called essential fats. They have the same status as vitamins and other essential nutrients in that without them in our diets we cannot live. They are particularly important for the developing baby and are used for brain, eye and nervous tissue development and to make sex hormones. They are also needed to reduce the risk of pre-eclampsia, pre-term and low birth weight babies, and may also help to stop the characteristic forgetfulness of pregnancy. We also need them to make substances called prostaglandins, which are hormone-like chemicals vital for a healthy pregnancy. These essential fats, and related fats, are linoleic acid (LA), gamma-linolenic acid (GLA), arachadonic acid (AA), eicosapentanoic acid (EPA) and decosahexanoic acid (DHA). Rather tellingly, the only time that the human body is able to make essential fats is when breast milk is produced, because the baby is unable to get them from any other source and will not thrive without them. If anything should underscore the importance of these fats to human survival, it is this fact. More of these fats are needed in the last trimester of pregnancy, and while breast-feeding. The best way to get these into the diet is to make sure that the fats you eat come from the foods already mentioned (seeds, nuts, oily fish and cold-pressed oils). A tablespoon of nutty-tasting flax seeds (grind them in a clean coffee grinder) added to cereals, yoghurt, soups or baking is a delicious way of getting the essential fats as well as a hefty dose of minerals and fibre.

Signs of insufficient levels of essential fats in the diet include dry skin, itchy skin, poor hair condition and brittle nails, dry eyes, stretch marks, eczema and other skin complaints. If you have any of these it would be worth taking a tablespoon of cold-pressed flax oil on your food daily (irrespective of the calories!) If you find that this is too much oil in one go, take half a tablespoonful twice a day on your food. Flax oil has a pleasant taste, but if you prefer you can mix it with olive oil, lemon, vinegar, honey or mustard to make a delicious salad or vegetable dressing.

sources of essential fats in the diet include

oily fish Eat oily fish such as mackerel, sardines, fresh tuna, salmon, pilchards, anchovies, shark, pink trout and halibut at least three times a week for maximum benefit.

fresh nuts They need to be fresh because the vital oils are denatured in hard or rancid nuts. Buying them shelled is fine, but keep them in the refrigerator to maintain freshness. Add, chopped, to all sorts of dishes, as well as snacking on them. Fresh nuts are also one of the best sources of vitamin E, and an excellent source of the fertility minerals zinc and selenium.

fresh seeds Add them whole, chopped or ground to a variety of dishes, including breakfast cereals, yoghurts and salads, as well using them in baking or just snacking on them. Include sunflower seeds, pumpkin seeds, sesame seeds and hemp seeds (not the smoking variety, but the munching variety!). Again, fresh seeds are superb sources of minerals for reproductive health.

dressings made with cold-pressed oils Store the oils in the refrigerator and do not allow them to go rancid. Use flax, sesame, walnut, sunflower and safflower. Extra-virgin olive oil does not contain the beneficial fats, but does have powerful and useful antioxidants and is ideal for mixing half-and-half with other oils to dress salads. Use olive oil to cook with but do not cook with the other oils as this destroys their benefits.

Calcium Rich Foods

3 servings daily of calcium rich foods (giving about 250 mg calcium each serving)

one serving is equal to:

200 ml/7 fl oz milk or yoghurt
45 g/1½ oz cheese
200 ml/7 fl oz calcium enriched soya milk or yoghurt
½ a 120 g can of sardines with the bones in or 1 250 g can of salmon
200 g/7 oz dark green leafy vegetables
a combination of 4 or 5 other high calcium foods, such as 25g/1 oz nuts or seeds, 1 orange, 85 g/3 oz kidney beans, 115 g/4 oz blackberries (see chart, page 73)

Calcium is essential during pregnancy to grow your baby's bones. If calcium is lacking from the diet it is leached from the mother's bones and teeth, and osteoporosis (mineral loss from bones) is fairly common in pregnancy. Most women recover this bone loss after pregnancy if their diet is rich in the necessary minerals, however hundreds of cases of fractures from osteoporosis are believed to happen each year and are often diagnosed incorrectly as back ache. This is likely to be worse if the mother has had eating disorders in the past, which is a strong risk factor for osteoporosis, making it more important than ever to eat well during pregnancy, breast-feeding and afterwards.

The advertised advantage of dairy produce is that it is a rich source of calcium. However, milk is a poor source of another essential mineral for bone health – magnesium. Several minerals work together to build healthy bones and of particular importance is the balance between calcium and magnesium. It is not enough to get sufficient calcium in the diet, you also need to be able to use it effectively in your bones. Magnesium allows the calcium to be correctly utilised and so foods that are rich in both of these minerals are better sources, overall, than foods that are rich in calcium but not in magnesium. The value of calcium from nuts, seeds and green leafy vegetables, therefore, as well as from fish bones (which are easy to eat when they have been softened by the canning process) is higher than that of the calcium from dairy produce. This is not to say that dairy produce has no value at all, just that it tends to be over-emphasised as a way of getting calcium. It is of far more value to achieve your daily calcium intake from a wide variety of foods, which give a good balance of minerals, and to top this up with some dairy produce.

From the point of view of general health, milk can tend to be 'mucus forming' for susceptible people, and it contributes to a wide variety of health problems such as rhinitis, hay fever, asthma, headaches, migraines, arthritis and digestive problems. Hard cheeses and yoghurt have a much better track record in not stimulating these responses, and these dairy products have just as high, if not higher, calcium values as milk. I would suggest limiting milk to that added to tea or used in cooking occasionally, and instead eating a portion of cheese or yoghurt daily and relying on getting the rest of your calcium intake from a wide variety of other foods such as dark green leafy vegetables, nuts, seeds and other foods (see page 73).

If you are eating dairy products, the most easily absorbable form is yoghurt. Because the proteins and milk sugars have been partially pre-digested by the bacteria used in the yoghurt-making process, yoghurt is generally more acceptable to human digestion than milk or cheese, the calcium is also more absorbable, and the B-vitamin levels have been improved.

One of the problems with dairy produce is that it can contribute a hefty number of calories to your daily intake. It is best, therefore, to concentrate on low fat versions, of which there are many choices. You can also cut back on creamy sauces and butter by using yoghurt when cooking or making salad dressings. Just mix some yoghurt with a little vinaigrette for an instant and delicious dressing. When cooking with yoghurt instead of cream, add it to the dish at the last minute otherwise it will curdle. Be cautious of 'low fat' dairy desserts, however, including fruit flavoured yoghurts, as these tend to be loaded with sugar or artificial sweeteners.

If you are avoiding dairy produce a good number of soya and other alternative milk products are fortified with calcium to mirror the mineral make-up of milk. Again, choose products with the minimum of added sugars. Remember that what you actually need is calcium and other minerals for bone health, not dairy produce. As long as you are eating a varied diet then you are probably getting sufficient calcium (see page 73 for sources of calcium).

Meat, Poultry, Fish, Eggs or Vegetarian Protein Sources

3–4 servings daily of meat, poultry, eggs or vegetarian protein sources (giving 20–25 g protein each)

one serving is equal to:

85 g/3 oz meat or poultry
100 g/4 oz fish
2 eggs plus 2 egg whites
100 g/4 oz cooked dried beans or peas
100 g/4 oz nuts
140 g/5 oz tofu (bean curd)
100 g/4 oz cheese

Proteins are the building blocks of life and it is vitally important that a pregnant woman gets sufficient protein to make her baby. Proteins are made up of molecular links called amino acids, and eight of these amino acids are essential for human health. We must get these amino acids from the diet as we are unable to fabricate them. All eight essential amino acids are present in animal foods, such as meat, poultry, fish, eggs and dairy produce, which makes these foods an easy way to get the proteins we need.

There are plenty of plant sources of these amino acids, but they do not, mostly, have the full complement of essential amino acids. Because of this, if you are a vegetarian, and particularly if you restrict dairy produce, it is important to get a wide variety of plant sources of proteins to make sure that you get the right balance. This means making sure that in the course of a day, you eat beans, pulses, grains, nuts and seeds.

At first glance it may seem that three or four portions of protein daily is a lot, however when you look at the portion sizes you will quickly realise that it is easy to overdo protein foods, and that is exactly what we tend to do, especially if we also drink a lot of milk or eat dairy products that are sources of protein as well as calcium. By the time you've had two eggs in an omelette for breakfast or lunch, and a hunk of cheese, some nuts and a yoghurt as snacks, you've almost had your quota for the day and you haven't even started on the meat yet! Pregnant women need more protein than normal, but only, on average, an extra 6 g. It is still important to limit the cow-size steaks, as having a large serving of meat is likely to mean that your vegetable intake is reduced – there simply isn't enough room on the plate for more food! The best way to make meat stretch further is to eat it as a small part of a larger meal. For instance, add it to stir-frys, use it as a topping for wholemeal pizzas, add to rice and vegetables used to stuff peppers and marrows, or to flavour bean stews. Red meat is an important source of iron and zinc, which are needed during pregnancy, but if you eat red meat, make sure that you trim all visible fat and that you skim off the fat from the top of casseroles and minced meat dishes (this is most easily done if you cool down the dish and skim off the hardened fat). The fat in meat is mostly saturated fat, and this can encourage inflammation and excessive weight gain.

Meat is generally high in saturated fats and has no fibre in it, while vegetarian sources of protein have virtually no saturated fats and are good sources of fibre. Because of this, favouring plant sources of protein is a clever thing to do a few times a week because the fibre helps to keep your digestive tract healthy, without contributing saturated fats to the diet. An excess of saturated fats in the diet is linked to a number of health problems, including inflammatory diseases such as arthritis and degenerative diseases such as heart disease and cancer. The animal sources of protein that are lowest in saturated fats are fish and game meat.

The oils found in oily fish, EPA and DHA, are particularly

beneficial during pregnancy. The placenta selectively absorbs these fats from the maternal bloodstream, and 18 per cent of the fats in the developing baby's brain are DHA. These fats are also essential for the development of the testes in male infants and for liver growth. Fish consumption over the last 50 years, however, has halved, and one fifth of people never eat oily fish at all. Ideally, you should eat it three times a week to gain the maximum benefit. Indeed, eating oily fish as a preferred source of protein instead of meat at least three times a week automatically redresses the balance in your diet away from saturated fats, towards the 'very long chain' unsaturated and valuable oils found in fish.

If you choose to avoid fish because you are a vegetarian, don't like it or are concerned about environmental toxins, then make sure you take flax oil or linseeds daily, as they will provide many of the same benefits. Toxins in fish have caused a lot of concern, but cooking reduces the levels and overall the benefits provided by the fats probably outweigh any possible dangers.

Fruit Feast

3–5 servings daily of fruit

one serving is equal to:

1 medium apple, orange, banana, peach, etc
2 kiwi fruits, 2 plums, 2 tangerines, etc
1 large slice melon, pineapple, etc
½ papaya, ½ grapefruit, ½ mango, etc
1 cup of grapes, cherries, raspberries, etc
150 ml/5 fl oz fruit juice

You really can't get enough fruit, and it is the ideal grab-and-eat snack. Three servings a day is the minimum to aim for, though five portions daily is much better. Fruit and vegetables are our most important sources of antioxidants. Fruit is also a valuable source of soluble fibre, and in addition helps keep calorie counts in a reasonable range. In fact, fruit fulfils the most important criteria for Eating for a Perfect Pregnancy – they are nutrient rich foods. Antioxidants are vital in the war that our bodies permanently wage with the outside world and they support the immune system as well as neutralise damaging free-radicals. Free-radicals are molecules that are 'loose cannons' and lead to oxidation damage which is linked to over 80 major human diseases. Recent research also suggests that antioxidants play a vital role in reducing the likelihood of you being one of the one-in-ten women who suffer pre-eclampsia during pregnancy (see **The Second Trimester**, page 161).

If plain fruit does not appeal all the time, ring the changes by making exotic fruit salads, fixing yourself a baked apple or banana, adding chopped fruit to yoghurt, or eating stewed fruit or dried fruit. You can also add fruit to salads and casseroles. Also, remember that a glass of orange or apple juice at breakfast counts towards your fruit intake. A terrific way of getting fruit into your diet is to whizz up milk shakes and smoothies using soft fruit such as peaches, ripe pears, bananas, kiwi, straw-berries, blackberries, mango, papaya, or any other soft fruit in season. Juices can be made from hard fruit, if you have a juicing machine, and pretty much anything can go in: apples, pine-apples, watermelon, harder pears or kiwi fruit, along with hard vegetables such as carrots, beetroot and green vegetables. If you are suffering from morning sickness, add a cube of ginger when you make your juice to help quell your queasiness.

Vegetable Variety

3–5 portions of vegetables daily

one serving is equal to:

75 g / 2½ oz of raw, leafy greens
100 g / 3½ oz of other vegetables (aim to eat at least one
     portion of yellow / orange vegetables – or fruit – daily)
150 ml / 5 fl oz glass of tomato or vegetable juice

Once again there really is no upper limit on the amount of mixed vegetables you can eat on a healthy diet; three servings daily is the minimum to aim for, five is ideal. Along with fruit they are a primary source of antioxidants and a valuable source of fibre. Ideally, one of your portions should be a dark green leafy vegetable, such as cabbage, kale, spinach or broccoli, as they are calcium and magnesium rich. Another portion of either vegetables or fruit should ideally be a yellow or orange option such as squash, pumpkin, orange / yellow peppers, carrots, cantaloupe, mango or apricots because they are particularly rich in beta-carotene and the other members of the carotenoid family, which are all potent antioxidants. These are highly beneficial in pregnancy for protecting both mother and baby. Vegetables are so versatile that increasing the number of vegetable dishes you eat shouldn't prove a problem. Choose fresh or frozen vegetables but avoid canned vegetables (other than canned beans, peas, tomatoes or carrots, which still have virtuous nutritional qualities, though wash off the salty water). Here are some ideas for delicious vegetables to add to your meals without resorting to over-boiled cabbage!

● Vegetable soups of all descriptions: spinach soup, tomato and basil soup, mixed vegetable soup, curried parsnip soup, lettuce and pea soup, gazpacho, beetroot soup, carrot and coriander soup.

● Adopt Mediterranean methods of preparing vegetables: ratatouille, vegetable sauces to use with pasta or rice (a sauce of aubergines, tomato, garlic and black olives is particularly delicious), grilled vegetables (peppers, fennel, courgettes and red onions), stuffed peppers, mushrooms in lemon, garlic and olive oil.

● Try some of the fabulous Indian vegetable dishes (just go easy on the ghee or oil): okra and onion, aubergine and tomato, spinach (sag) bahji.

● See how creative you can get with salads: green bean, tomato and red onion, salad Niçoise, three colour grated salad (carrot, beet and fennel), courgette, tomato, spring onion and black olives.

● Go Eastern and make stir-frys with any number of ingredients: bean sprouts, carrot slivers, spring onions, peppers, slivered cabbage, baby corn, broccoli in black bean sauce.

● Make vegetable dips such as tomato, green pepper and onion salsa, aubergine dip, or chickpea dip to eat with hot wholemeal pitta bread or vegetable sticks.

Bread, Cereals, Rice, Pasta, Potatoes

6–9 portions of carbohydrate foods daily

one serving is equal to:

1 slice of bread, ½ a bun, ½ bagel or ½ muffin
25 g/1 oz dry cereal
50–100g/2–4 oz cooked cereal, rice or pasta
1 medium potato

Carbohydrate foods are our main source of energy, and you

need plenty of that when you are pregnant! They also provide fibre, when they are eaten as wholegrains, which is vital for regulating bowels. When Eating for a Perfect Pregnancy it is really important to eat all of your grains, whether rice, bread, pasta or cereals, in their wholegrain form if you and your baby are to get the maximum number of nutrients and the most fibre from them. This means eating foods such as wholemeal bread, brown rice, rye bread, rye crackers, whole oats and jacket potatoes. The refining process strips grains of between 60–90 per cent of the minerals they contain, and, nutritionally speaking, refined grains are poor relatives of whole grains. Even if the bread or cereal packet proclaims it is 'enriched with X different vitamins and minerals' it will still be devoid of a range of other vitamins and minerals, such as selenium, chromium, manganese and magnesium, which make unprocessed grains so useful in the diet.

If you find that some grains do not agree with you (as is common with wheat), and you have been avoiding them because they cause symptoms such as bloating, flatulence, skin conditions or headaches, there are other grains and starches that you should be able to eat quite comfortably. Some options to experiment with include: oats, rye, barley, rice, millet, buckwheat, corn, quinoa or spelt. By including these other grains in your diet you can get the widest variety of nutrients. Think laterally when you are making dishes. For instance, if you always include rice with a particular dish, experiment with using barley, millet or buckwheat instead. Substitute some of the flour in baking recipes with other flours, such as maize, buckwheat or oat flour. There are also many starchy alternatives to grains that are satisfying and interesting accompaniments to a meal. Apart from the familiar, and versatile, potato, you could flirt with sweet potatoes and yams (both extremely high in beta-carotene), breadfruit, sago (made from the pith of palms) or tapioca (made from cassava). The real point of this is to experiment with a varied and interesting diet – later on your baby may also benefit, once born, by enjoying a more varied choice of foods when you are weaning her or him.

Putting It All Together

Well, that's the theory. So how do you make it work? You could keep a picture of the pyramid in your mind and as you eat throughout the day you could mentally cross off what fulfils the 'contract'. If you are not great at visualisation you could keep a little tick list and cross off the food groupings on paper. Another way is to work out an eating plan that more or less fits in with the plan overleaf, but filling in foods and ideas that you enjoy. Remember that variety is the most important thing and if you choose cereal one morning for breakfast, choose a different cereal or toast using a different grain the next day. So if, for instance, you have wholemeal toast one morning, have rye toast the next, porridge the day after and brown rice puffs after that – this will give you a wide variety of nutrients. It is probably easiest to write down five breakfasts you enjoy, ten fast meal options and at least ten main meals and to keep rotating them and changing the focus by using different vegetables or fruit in season. Once you get the hang of it you will be able to be very flexible and successfully Eat for a Perfect Pregnancy.

MEAL	SERVING	FOOD SUGGESTION
Breakfast	cereals or starches (2)	50 g/2 oz muesli, 25 g/1 oz seeds
	calcium rich food	calcium enriched soya milk or dairy milk
	fruit portions (2)	chopped fruit on the muesli and a glass of fresh juice
Snack	fruit portion	sliced strawberries on
	cereals or starches	oat cakes
Lunch	protein/essential fats	salmon with ginger and lemon grass
	calcium rich food/vegetable	stir-fried broccoli
	yellow/orange vegetable	with carrot sticks (and onions, garlic, etc)
	cereals or starches	baby potatoes or quinoa

(these could be combined to make a cold dish to eat at work)

Snack	protein (½ portion)	fresh nuts
	fruit portion	dried apple rings
Evening	protein & vegetable	chickpeas, spinach and onion bake
	calcium rich food/protein	45 g/1½ oz grated cheese topping
	cereals or starches (2)	brown rice

BEYOND THE PYRAMID

The pyramid represents an easy way to evaluate your daily intake of food, to provide the most important nutrients for your pregnancy. By visualising where the food groups appear on the pyramid you can readily work out if your meal, or indeed your whole day of eating, more or less fits into the pyramid.

But of course many other factors influence our daily intake of nutrients – what we drink, fibre in the diet, if we are vegetarians and so on. Let's take a look beyond the pyramid.

Liquid Refreshment

Drinking plenty of water is essential for your baby, and for you. Your baby is made up of 70 per cent water and needs water just as much as proteins and fats to build up tissues, organs and the brain. You will also benefit hugely from drinking water, as it helps to alleviate, or avoid altogether, a host of problems that can be worsened by pregnancy – constipation, dry skin complaints and urinary tract infections such as cystitis.

Two litres/3½ pints of water a day is a good maintenance amount to drink, but you may need to increase this to 3 litres/5¼ pints daily when you are breast-feeding. Find a way to remind yourself to drink your water – set a timer every hour to drink a glass, or make a point of drinking a glass before each meal, and one after, or keep a 2-litre bottle by your desk and sip it all day long. It doesn't matter how you achieve it, just make sure that by hook, or by crook, you drink enough water.

Do not be tempted to substitute caffeinated drinks for your water allocation. Caffeine dehydrates the body and causes water-*loss*. The more you drink coffee, tea or colas the more water you lose.

If you get bored with the idea of plain water, there are many ways it can be jazzed up: drink hot water with a squeeze of lemon and a little honey, keep a jug of fruit tea in the refrigerator topped up with fruit slices and mint or make your own cordial with 80 per cent fruit (such as berries) and 20 per cent fructose (fruit sugar is available from health food shops and is a better alternative to white or brown sugar) and dilute as you would other cordials. Other drinks that nourish you are fresh fruit or vegetable juices that you can dress up – for instance make yourself a non-alcoholic fruit punch or a spicy virgin Mary.

Fibre Facts

When you follow **The Food Pyramid** plan (see page 50), you will get the necessary 25 g of fibre a day to keep your digestive tract healthy. Pregnancy is a time when the digestive tract slows down slightly and keeping fibre levels topped up helps to avoid constipation. One of the worst ways to get more fibre into your diet is to buy wheatbran and add it liberally to your foods. This fibre can be extremely irritating to the inner wall of the digestive tract and is also notorious for reducing the absorption of minerals (see **Nutrient Robbers**, page 71). It is far better to increase your fibre levels by eating more foods rich in gentle fibres, which will bulk out the stools more effectively. Beans, pulses, peas, porridge oats, fruit and vegetables are all excellent sources of fibre.

As well as keeping you 'moving', fibre helps to keep the bacteria in the bowels in a healthy balance. These bacteria can be highly beneficial if they are in the right balance and, amongst other jobs, they help to make a significant number of the B-vitamins, including folic acid and vitamin K. Vitamin K is needed to ensure healthy clotting of blood, and boosting levels helps to reduce the chance of a lot of blood loss at birth. All parents are offered a vitamin K injection, or drops, for their baby when they are born to avoid problems with haemorrhagic disease (a bleeding disorder). Boosting your fibre levels to ensure that you are making more vitamin K can only be beneficial.

Nutrient Paupers

One pretty good philosophy to follow when buying food is 'If you don't recognise the ingredients on the package as food, don't buy it'. This rule gets rid of a vast number of fillers, additives, colours and flavourings. With the possible exception of some antioxidants and preservatives, these additives are unnecessary, and contravene the first rule of Eating for a Perfect Pregnancy. They do not add any nutritional value, and more often than not mask cheap, nutrient depleted, highly processed ingredients. The unpalatable truth about convenience foods is that they are styled to suit the manufacturers and not us. There are three major problems with mass-produced convenience foods:

- They tend to use fillers such as the refined starch maltodextrine, which glue the products together and are extremely cheap, but they have little or no nutritional value. Often these fillers are added because they can carry a lot of water – the cheapest ingredient of all. If you fill up on foods containing these ingredients, you are eating a nutrient-poor diet, which is the exact opposite of what you need to be doing in pregnancy.
- Eighty per cent of the sugar and salt we consume comes from convenience and packaged foods. The manufacturers claim that it is consumer demand that keeps levels high, but the reality is that these are highly addictive ingredients that make people crave more. They are also taste-bud blunters and thus allow large amounts of fillers and fats, including hydrogenated fats, to be used – fat on its own

does not taste very good, but add sugar and salt and you can use much more.

● Even when foods say they are fortified with nutrients they are still nutrient paupers. The government requires white flour, for instance, to be fortified with B-vitamins, calcium and iron to make up for nutrients lost in the refining process. However, there are many other nutrients, which are intrinsic to the whole grain, that are not added back.

processed and convenience foods to avoid or reduce drastically

● packet mixes (i.e. cake mixes or instant puddings)
● canned foods (apart from canned fish, tomatoes, beans)
● deep-fried foods
● pies and pasties
● most commercially made cakes and biscuits (there are some exceptions)
● sugary foods
● artificially sweetened foods and drinks
● colas, sodas and squashes (including low calorie, low sugar varieties)

It is difficult to avoid packaged foods altogether, but it helps to be more selective and to read the labels. Not all packaged foods are terrible and if you learn to make informed choices, you will win. Select good quality rye crackers or oatcakes instead of water biscuits. Choose sun dried tomatoes or olives in olive oil instead of canned vegetables. Pick fruit juices instead of fruit squashes. Mix fresh fruit with live yoghurt instead of buying highly sweetened novelty yoghurts, fromage frais or creamy desserts. Eat, in moderation, wholemeal biscuits, fruit filled biscuits (such as fig rolls), fruit juice sweetened bran muffins or oat flapjacks instead of most other biscuits, doughnuts and cakes. They may all be fairly high in sugar, but at least they provide a reasonable dose of nutrients and fibre as well.

Nutrient Robbers

When Eating for a Perfect Pregnancy not only do you need to eat foods that are nutrient-dense rather than nutrient-poor, you also need to avoid substances that actively rob your body of nutrients. This is not quite as daunting as it sounds, because one way or another we have already covered a lot of what you need to do. The following is just a summary of what these nutrient-robbers are and how they do their dastardly work.

The most damaging anti-nutrients are alcohol and cigarettes. Apart from contributing damaging chemicals, they also deplete the body of nutrients. Sugar is another culprit, and also one of the most damaging sources of empty calories. Not only does sugar not contribute anything, it also causes fluctuations in blood sugar which leads to damaged body tissues, which in turn uses up valuable antioxidants. Sugar also causes a net loss of the mineral chromium, which is needed to metabolise it, and once used needs to be replaced from the diet. Sugar is ubiquitous in our food supply, and one of the aims of Eating for a Perfect Pregnancy is to dramatically reduce the typical daily intake of sugar and replace it with fibre-rich foods such as fruit, vegetables and wholegrains which help to stabilise blood sugar and provide nutrients such as chromium.

There are other anti-nutrients which are just as important but not as obvious as sugar, alcohol or cigarettes. As it happens, smoking is one of the main sources of this deadly duo – cadmium and lead. One of the ways in which these heavy metals cause problems is to actively interfere with the uptake of nutritional minerals from food such as zinc and iron. Conversely, if you are on a zinc and iron rich diet this will minimise the effect that these heavy metals can have. Calcium, magnesium, selenium and vitamin C rich foods are also all good at getting rid of heavy metals from the body.

The caffeine in coffee, tea and colas will reduce the intake of nutrients from a meal, but the tannins in tea can also have a bad effect as they interfere with iron uptake from food by up to 70 per cent. So if you have to have a cup of tea it is best to not take it immediately after a meal when it can be most disruptive. Better to have hot water with a slice of lemon, and save your tea for in between meals.

Even some seemingly benign foods, which can be considered healthy in most respects, can act as anti-nutrients if they are eaten in disproportionately large amounts. This is because they contain high amounts of phytates and oxalates. Phytates found in wheat bran can limit the uptake of minerals (such as calcium, iron and zinc) from meals and this is best resolved by concentrating on other wholegrains which do not have the same effect. Porridge oats, muesli made with a variety of grains (such as oat, millet and buckwheat flakes with nuts, seeds and fruit), or corn-flake type cereals made from quinoa, amranth and millet flakes are all good options. If you are a very keen vegetable eater and find that you are eating a high proportion of dark green leafy vegetables you may need to be aware that substances called oxalates found in vegetables such as spinach and kale can limit mineral absorption from meals, particularly iron, so while dark green leafy vegetables are healthy on many fronts, it is best to vary your intake.

VITAMINS AND MINERALS NEEDED FOR A HEALTHY PREGNANCY

There are around 13 essential vitamins and 20 essential minerals that we must get from our food. Deficiencies of any of these nutrients can have an adverse effect both on the development of a baby, and in the fertility of the parents in the first place. Let's look at the most important nutrients for growing a healthy baby.

The Calcium Question and Other Nutrients for Bone Health – Magnesium and Vitamin D

Apart from bone and tooth health, calcium is needed for all nerve impulses and for blood clotting. The UK RNI (recommended nutrient intake) for calcium is 700 mg daily for both non-pregnant and pregnant women. The US RDA (recommended daily allowance) is 700 mg for non-pregnant women and 1,200 mg daily for pregnant and breast-feeding women. So, as you can see, there is already confusion about how much women should obtain from their diet. Luckily, nature is cleverer than humans at determining what a woman needs. Calcium absorption from the diet increases in pregnant women to about 70 per cent of the calcium ingested, against the usual amount of around 25 per cent.

Food portions	Calcium (mg)
whitebait (100 g)	850
milk, semi-skimmed (300 ml)	350
Cheddar/Edam (50 g)	350
sardines (70 g)	350
pinto beans, cooked (200 g)	250
enriched flour (100 g)	200
spring greens, spinach, raw (100 g)	180
tofu, calcium enriched (100g)	180
sesame seeds (20 g)	150

Food portions	Calcium (mg)
prawns (80 g)	120
baked beans (200 g)	100
pilchards, canned (100 g)	100
chickpeas (150 g)	100
salmon, canned (120 g)	100
molasses (25 g)	100
oranges, 1 large	70
bread, 2 slices any type	70
almonds, 20 shelled	50
dried fruit – dates, raisins, figs (35 g)	25
eggs, 1 large	25
carrot, 1 medium	25
cabbage, leeks, green beans (50 g)	25

If you generally avoid dairy produce, remember that this is fine as long as you are eating a varied diet consisting of plenty of other sources of calcium. Remember, too, that calcium from sources other than dairy, particularly from nuts, seeds, green leafy vegetables and canned fish, has a good proportion of magnesium, which further improves the usage of calcium. The UK RNI for magnesium is 270 mg. Magnesium is needed to make new tissue, both maternal and foetal, is used for more than 300 different enzyme processes and is linked to a lower risk of pre-eclampsia, premature babies, low birth weight babies and higher Apgar tests (a test which is used to measure the initial health of a baby).

Food portions	Magnesium (mg)
millet, cooked (230 g)	350
lima (butter) beans, black-eyed peas (170 g)	100
muesli, 1 bowl (100 g)	90
All-bran (50 g)	90

Food portions	Magnesium (mg)
Brazil nuts, 10 shelled	90
peanuts, 30	60
rice, brown boiled (150 g)	60
baked beans (200 g)	60
bread, 2 slices, wholemeal	60
carrot juice (300 ml)	50
almonds, 10 shelled	50
hazelnuts, 30 shelled	50
Weetabix, 2	50
prawns, cooked (80 g)	50
yoghurt, low fat (300 ml)	40
milk, semi-skimmed (300 ml)	20

Another mineral needed to balance calcium and for bone health is phosphorus and the UK RNI for pregnant women for this is 550 mg. Phosphorus is so widely distributed in foods that there is no need to even think about low levels. On the other hand, cola-type drinks have excessively high levels which can have a negative impact by unbalancing calcium levels and causing calcium to be excreted. Colas are thought to be one of the reasons why teenage girls are now showing signs of osteoporosis, and are therefore unlikely to be beneficial for a baby's growing bones.

Calcium absorption into the bones is also improved by vitamin D. Ensure that you get some sun (half an hour on average for medium tone Caucasian skins, is sufficient for your skin to manufacture vitamin D, but not enough to burn if you avoid the hottest part of the day) and that you eat oily fish, eggs and fortified cereals to maximise your body's ability to use calcium. The RNI for pregnant women is 400 ius (10 mcg/μg) daily. A supplement which contains more than 400 ius (10 mcg/μg) of vitamin D is not advised as an excess of vitamin D can be toxic to a developing baby.

Food portions	Vitamin D iu/mcg (µg)
Oily fish such as mackerel, herrings, kippers (110 g)	800/20
salmon, canned (100 g)	500/12.5
sardines, tuna, canned (100 g)	200/5
egg, 1 medium	40/1
bran based breakfast cereals, such as bran flakes and All-bran (40 g)	30/0.8
whole and semi-skimmed milk, liver, some cheeses, ice cream	small amounts
(note in the USA milk is enriched with vitamin D)	

Stay in the Pink – with Zinc!

Zinc is vital for all aspects of pregnancy. It is needed for sperm and egg growth, for fertilisation, brain and immune system development, and for the baby to mature in most other respects. The reason for this is that zinc, together with the vitamin that works alongside it, vitamin B6, is used for every stage of protein synthesis by the DNA of cells – in other words for the growth and repair of tissues. In particular, deficiencies of zinc are related to low birth weight babies, as well as to the incidence of cleft palates and hare lips. Interestingly, boy babies use up more zinc than girl babies. One of the typical signs of reduced levels of zinc is stretch marks on the skin, and so making sure you have enough zinc is one way of reducing the likelihood of developing them. Zinc is also one of the best protectors against lead pollution, which can adversely affect a developing baby.

The UK RNI for zinc for a pregnant woman is 7 mg daily, but this is probably an extremely conservative amount and the diets of many people, 31 per cent in fact, are deficient of even this amount. An optional intake of 15–20 mg is probably more suited to pregnancy. If you are going to supplement zinc I would suggest between 10–15 mg daily as a good level, along with 1 mg of copper for each 10 mg of zinc, to keep these two minerals in balance. The UK RNI for breast-feeding women is 13 mg.

Food portions	Zinc (mg)
oysters, 1 dozen raw	80
popcorn (100 g)	8
sesame seeds (100 g)	8
beef, cooked (100 g)	5
crab, cooked (100 g)	5
All-bran (50 g)	2.5
lobster, cooked (80 g)	2.5
walnuts, shelled (100 g)	2.5
muesli (100 g)	2.5
sardines, canned (70 g)	2.5
chickpeas, cooked (150 g)	1.5
bran flakes (50 g)	1.5
Cheddar (50 g)	1.5
bread, wholemeal, 2 slices	1.5
pasta, wholemeal (150 g)	1
Brazil nuts, 10 shelled	1
peanuts, shelled (25 g)	1
Weetabix, 2	1
soya beans, cooked (100 g)	1
pulses (100 g)	1
baked beans (200 g)	1

Iron Rations

Iron is the mineral needed to make red blood cells, and it is responsible for making the oxygen carrying component, haemo-globin. Iron absorption increases during pregnancy, so as long as you are not anaemic in the first place you should be OK.

However, this vital mineral is sufficiently low in the female population – 89 per cent get less than the 14.8 mg UK RNI – to account for one in six women of child-bearing age being either anaemic, or having a borderline low level. Because women lose blood when they menstruate this leaves them susceptible to excessive iron loss, which may compound a diet which is also deficient in this mineral. Until recently, it was common for women to be given iron routinely during their pregnancy to avoid anaemia (see **Anaemia**, page 159). This is no longer the case, however, because there is a realisation that it is not always needed.

If you have to take an iron supplement from your doctor, take it separately from other supplements to improve absorption (and take with orange juice). An organic iron supplement such as iron ascorbate can be taken with other supplements. A pre-natal formula that gives you 10–15 mg of iron daily is fine to take in general, but if you are diagnosed with anaemia by your doctor you may need to take up to 40 mg.

Food portions	Iron (mg)
cockles, cooked (100 g)	20
bran flakes (50 g)	8.5
potato flour (50 g)	8.5
liver, cooked (100 g)	8.5
soya flour (100 g)	8.5
spirulina (25 g)	7
pumpkin seeds (50 g)	7
mussels, cooked (80 g)	6
beef, cooked (150 g)	5
chickpeas, cooked (150 g)	5
apricots, dried (100 g)	5
baked beans (12 oz)	5
molasses (30 g)	5

Food portions	Iron (mg)
Jerusalem artichokes (100 g)	3
soya beans, cooked (100 g)	3
tofu (100 g)	3
corned beef (100 g)	3
pilchards, canned (100 g)	2.5
lentils (150 g)	2.5
figs, 4 dried	2.5
cocoa powder (25 g)	2.5
kidney beans, cooked (100 g)	1.8
soya milk (300 ml)	1.8

The Antioxidant Nutrients

The antioxidant nutrients are principally vitamins A, C, E and the mineral selenium. There are many hundreds of other antioxidant nutrients in food, which include the carotenes, quercitin, flavanoids and phenols. The second lot of antioxidants are not considered vital for life – in other words there is no deficiency disease associated with not having specific nutrients. A diet rich in fruit and vegetables, however, which provides these compounds is indisputably the most protective type of diet against a wide variety of diseases. Eating fruit and vegetables is also one of the greatest gifts you can give your developing baby.

Here we will concentrate on the specific antioxidant nutrients which are known to affect the outcome of pregnancy positively. All the antioxidants work together, and while it is useful to have, say, a good intake of vitamin C, it will work much more powerfully if it is eaten as part of a varied diet rich in the other antioxidants.

Vitamin C is necessary for so many functions in the human body they are almost too numerous to list – building white blood cells, building collagen (including a strong membrane around the baby), strengthening arteries, protecting gums, building healthy bones, making energy in each and every cell, and, of course, acting as an antioxidant. The RNI is a paltry 40 mg daily (50 mg in the last trimester). This is equivalent to the amount you get in one orange or a portion of cauliflower. The US figures for vitamin C have just been revised upwards, and I firmly believe that the RNI needs to be at least 200 mg, or the amount you would get from about six to eight portions of fruit and vegetables. It is perfectly safe to supplement one gram of vitamin C in pregnancy, and there are many reasons for doing so, including reducing the risk of pre-eclampsia, maintaining healthy gums and avoiding varicose veins. If you are going to take a vitamin C supplement, it is best to take a non-acidic version, such as magnesium ascorbate or potassium ascorbate, which avoids the very slight potential for it to upset your stomach, and to take one with bioflavonoids. The only people who should not take vitamin C are those who have been diagnosed with a condition called haemachromatosis, where you have an excess of iron in the blood, which can be made worse by taking vitamin C. Reports about vitamin C increasing the risk of kidney stones are inaccurate.

Food portions	Vitamin C (mg)
guava (100 g)	230
peppers, red or green (50 g)	130
Brussel sprouts, cooked (100 g)	110
blackcurrants, stewed (100 g)	110
kiwi fruit, raw (100 g)	90
papaya, 1 slice	90
orange juice, one large glass (200ml)	80
mango, one medium	50
cabbage, raw (100 g)	50
lychees (100 g)	50

Food portions	Vitamin C (mg)
broccoli, cooked (100 g)	50
cauliflower, cooked (100 g)	50
tangerines, 2	50
tomatoes, 2	50
peach, 1 medium	30
mangetout (50 g)	30
sweet potato, cooked (150 g)	30
cabbage, boiled (100 g)	20
passion fruit, 4	20

Vitamin A is needed for foetal lung and kidney development. While dietary sources of vitamin A are fine in pregnancy (other than liver which needs to be limited – see page 103), supplements containing more than 5,000 ius/1500 mcg (µg) vitamin A are not advised (see page 22). Because vitamin A is fat soluble it can build up in the body to toxic levels which might affect the developing baby. Beta-carotene is a member of the carotenoid family of antioxidant compounds which are found in most yellow/orange foods and in dark green leafy vegetables. Because beta-carotene converts into vitamin A, it is advised that any supplements are mainly based on beta-carotene. This is because it is not stored and any excess can be excreted harmlessly in the urine.

Some people do not make the conversion from beta-carotene to vitamin A very well and these are principally those with diabetes or an underactive thyroid. This does not mean that these people should take more vitamin A during pregnancy, but it does mean that they need to keep their insulin or thyroid hormone levels regulated by whichever method is advised by their doctor.

Food portion	Vitamin A iu/mcg (µg)
liver, calves', cooked (90 g)	36,000 /120,000
cod liver oil (10 ml)	1,800 /6000
liver sausage (35 g)	870 / 2900
cornmeal	550 /1800
cream, double or whipping (35 g)	190 /650
Cheddar (50 g)	150/500
whole milk (300 ml)	150/500
Brie (50 g)	150/500
egg, 1 medium	100/330
cream, single (35 g)	100/330
butter (10 g)	80/270
margarine, fortified (10 g)	80/270
kidney, lamb's, cooked (75 g)	80/270
herring, cooked (100 g)	60/200
mackerel, cooked (100 g)	60/200
yoghurt, whole milk (150 g)	40/130
taramasalata (100 g)	40/130

The chemical name for vitamin E is tocopherol, which comes from the Greek meaning 'to give birth'. This is because vitamin E is recognised as being vital for a healthy live birth. Rats deprived of vitamin E quickly become unable to reproduce, and in humans increasing vitamin E has been linked to a lower risk of miscarriage. Natural vitamin E is also known to help red blood cells survive in premature babies and avoid foetal oxygen deficiency. Vitamin E is a valuable antioxidant and on a processed food diet is quite difficult to get, especially as it is stripped out of grains in the refining process. The levels that have been associated with giving protection from the risk of pre-eclampsia (see page 161) are far in excess of the amount that anyone could get from their diet. To get just 150 ius/100 mg of vitamin E you would need to eat one of the following: 1,400 slices of wholemeal bread; 850 bowls of cornflakes; 180 boiled eggs; 9 kg boiled spinach; 15 kg peanuts; or 200 ml of sunflower oil. Vitamin E is very safe to supplement at around 400 ius/270 mg, though, as it acts as a blood thinning agent, it should be taken only with professional advice by anyone who is already on blood thinning medication such as Warfarin. It may be a good idea to lower the dose of any supplement to 100 ius a couple of weeks before the anticipated birth to reduce the chance of excess bleeding during labour, though this is a theoretical hazard rather than a likely one. If you take supplements you must make sure that they are d-alpha-tocopherol, which is the natural form of vitamin E that has been shown to be active in the placenta, rather than dl-alpha-tocopherol, which includes an unnatural form that has been shown to be of much less value when compared to the natural form. The labels on supplement bottles will usually say 'natural' or 'natural source' vitamin E, and if they do not then assume that they use the synthetic compound.

Food sources	Vitamin E (ius/mg)
wheatgerm oil (1 tbsp)	40/27
soyabean oil (1 tbsp)	18/12
almonds (50 g)	18/12
sunflower oil (1 tbsp)	15/10
walnuts, shelled (50 g)	15/10
lima (butter) beans, cooked (100 g)	10.5/7
sunflower seeds (1 tbsp)	10.5/7
sweet potatoes, boiled (150 g)	10.5/7
cashews, dry roasted (50 g)	7.5/5
flour, wholewheat (100 g)	5.5/3.5
wheatgerm, 2 heaped tbsp	5.5/3.5
peanuts, 30	5.5/3.5
avocado pear, 1/2	5.5/3.5
rice, brown, cooked (100 g)	3/2

Food sources	Vitamin E (ius/mg)
blackberries, stewed (100 g)	3/2
tomatoes, 2	3/2
chickpeas, cooked (100 g)	2.5/1.5
bread, wholemeal, 2 slices	2.5/1.5
salmon, canned (100 g)	2.5/1.5
olive oil, 1 tbsp	1.5/1

Selenium is the antioxidant mineral needed for the main anti-oxidant and detoxification enzymes which we make. The UK RNI for selenium is 60 mcg, yet about half the population does not get this amount, because the soil in which most of our grains are grown are depleted of this mineral. Selenium can be toxic in high amounts and for this reason supplementation over 200 mcg daily is unwise. In pregnancy, to be on the safe side, supplementation should probably not exceed 100 mcg. Seafood is a good source of selenium and if you follow the recommendations to eat fish regularly this can help to boost levels from the diet.

Food portions	Selenium mcg (μg)
brazil nuts, 10	200
clams, raw (180 g)	100
cashews, dry roasted (100 g)	65
prawns (100 g)	40
white fish, cooked (150 g)	40
wholemeal bread, 2 slices	30
molasses, blackstrap (25 g)	30
pork (100 g)	15
mushrooms, cooked (70 g)	8
chicken, skinless (100 g)	8
pulses (100 g)	4
baked beans (200 g)	4

Food portions	Selenium mcg (µg)
egg, I	3–25 (depending on how the chicken is fed)
courgettes, cabbage, carrots, orange, banana, green vegetables	2 per 100 g of food
peanuts, 30	I
almonds, 20	I

B-Vital with B-Vitamins

The B-vitamins are essential for energy production and metabolism, for cell division, brain development and to make blood cells. They are water soluble nutrients, which means that it is necessary to get a fresh supply of B-vitamins daily to maintain body functions. There are several members of the B-vitamin complex and they all work better together. Taking too much of one B-vitamin can imbalance the effects of others. Folic acid is a member of this group of vitamins and it is now considered absolutely necessary to supplement before, and during, the first three months of pregnancy if you wish to dramatically reduce the risk (by 75 per cent) of having a child with spina bifida or other neural tube defects. However, of those women that are aware of this fact 70 per cent still do not take folic acid before conception. Nevertheless, the awareness that there is has had a huge impact and cut the incidence of neural tube defects from 4 in 1,000 in the 1970s to 0.3 in 1,000 today.

The only problem with supplementing folic acid on its own is that it can mask deficiencies of other B-vitamins and it certainly works better with the others. I would therefore recommend taking a B-complex supplement that includes the whole family rather than just folic acid in isolation, to get the best effect. Choose a supplement with 400 mcg of folic acid and 25–50 mg of most of the other B-vitamins (25 mcg of B12). It is suggested that the 25 per cent of cases of spina bifida that are resistant to folic acid alone may respond to folic acid taken in conjunction with inisitol (another B vitamin) and B12.

B Vitamin	Found in
B1 (thiamin)	whole wheat, brown rice, brewer's yeast, pork, whitebait, beef, brazil nuts, peanuts, kidney beans, oranges
B2 (riboflavin)	liver, whole wheat, brown rice, soya milk, Marmite, duck, cottage cheese, pinto beans, yoghurt, mackerel, mushrooms, eggs, sesame seeds, asparagus
B3 (niacin)	liver, tuna (canned), chicken, lamb's kidneys, fish, pork, wheatgerm, mackerel, peanuts, sardines, black beans, peaches, pinto beans, whole wheat, Marmite, brown rice, semi-skimmed or skimmed milk, baked beans, peas, chickpeas, tomato juice
B5 (pantothenic acid)	peanuts, liver, lamb's kidneys, avocado, hazelnuts, mushrooms, chicken, sunflower seeds, whole grains, pumpkin, eggs, semi-skimmed or skimmed milk, dates, cottage cheese, potatoes, yoghurt, lentils, bananas
B6 (pyridoxine)	whole grains, sunflower seeds, lentils, potatoes, white fish, kidney beans, avocado, liver, tuna (canned), sweet potato, banana, baked beans, peanuts, pork, cashews, brewer's yeast, soya milk, milk (any)
B12 (cobalamin)	clams, liver, kidneys, mackerel fillets, pilchards, sardines, tuna, meat, white fish, soya milk, eggs, pork, milk (any), cheese, fortified cereals, Marmite, yoghurt

B Vitamin	Found in
folic acid	brewer's yeast, liver, spinach, potatoes, endive (chicory), Brussel sprouts, oranges and orange juice, whole grains, fortified cereals, chickpeas, asparagus, kale, broccoli, mung beans, black-eyed beans, lamb's kidneys, pistachio nuts, cabbage, peas, okra, soya milk, cauliflower, Marmite

Iodine Intake

This trace mineral is needed to maintain thyroid function and optimise metabolism, which is necessary for normal development of the baby's brain and central nervous system. It is rich in all seafood and sea vegetables, and if you are following the recommendation to regularly include fish in your diet you should get sufficient iodine. Some prenatal formulas will include around 40 mcg (µg) in their formulation. The UK RNI is 140 mcg (µg) daily, while the 'Eurodiet' goals are probably about to be set at 200 mcg for pregnant women. Iodised salt is widely available, but if you are keeping your salt intake to a moderate level by not adding it to your cooking, you will need to get iodine from elsewhere. Kelp is the richest source of iodine at 550 mcg (µg) per gram of kelp. A tasty alternative to salt is to use kelp granules (available from health food shops) in your grinder and add a sprinkling to all savoury dishes.

Food sources	Iodine mcg (µg)
haddock, cooked (150 g)	300
mackerel, cooked (150 g)	200
cod, cooked (150 g)	150
yoghurt (150 g)	90
pilchards, canned in tomato (100 g)	50

Food sources	Iodine mcg (μg)
plaice, cooked (150 g)	50
hard cheese (50 g)	25
corned beef, canned (100 g)	14
chicken, skinless (100 g)	5

Chromium Curbs Cravings

This mineral is used by the body to help regulate blood sugar balance and it is the core mineral for a substance we produce called glucose tolerance factor. People who are deficient in chromium often have a problem regulating their blood sugar levels and this can lead to sugar and other carbohydrate cravings. Only one in ten people consume enough chromium and breast-feeding lowers body stores of this mineral. There is no RNI for chromium but government health information notes that 25 mcg is probably a reasonable minimum. Supplements contain between 50–200 mcg, which is perfectly safe in pregnancy. The only people who may need to treat this level with caution are insulin dependent diabetics, because chromium makes insulin more effective. Foods which are rich in this mineral include shellfish, chicken, brewer's yeast, brown rice, rye bread, whole wheat, cooked dried beans, liver, eggs, bananas, carrots, lettuce, cabbage, broccoli, wheatgerm, oranges, green beans, mushrooms, spinach, orange juice, apples and potatoes.

VEGETARIAN AND VEGAN MOTHERS

Vegetarians of every type and description have been having healthy babies throughout history, and as long as you are well nourished and eating a healthy vegetarian diet there is no cause for concern, and certainly no need to compromise on any ethical views you may have on the subject. Nevertheless, it pays to acquaint yourself with how you can ensure that you get all the nutrients you need.

Is the vegetarian diet the healthiest option all round? There is no completely straightforward answer to this question. Certainly, we are aware that a diet high in saturated fats and low in fibre, which is typical of high meat and dairy food diets, is linked to a greater risk of heart disease, cancer and arthritis. But the key word here is excess. The detrimental effects of a meat eating diet, and the beneficial effects of a vegetarian diet on these diseases may actually be linked to the inclusion or absence of fruit, vegetables and other fibre rich foods such as pulses and grains, rather than eating animal protein per se. It seems that most of the protective effect comes from eating a high amount of plant foods and oils such as olive oil, rather than from avoiding meat totally. Meat is a source of highly absorbable forms of certain minerals, such as iron and zinc, which are often deficient in the diet. These nutrients, and others, can all be obtained from a vegetarian diet, but attention needs to be paid to ensuring that the diet is not deficient in any way. Probably the most common mistake made when someone decides to become a vegetarian, is that they simply give up meat and do not increase their intake of suitable substitutes. It is just as easy to be a junk-food vegetarian as it is to be a junk-food meat eater! A regime of doughnuts, chips and chocolate is a vegetarian one, but not a healthy one.

Women who eat eggs and dairy (and sometimes those who call themselves vegetarian also eat fish) can pretty much follow the diet suggestions covered in this chapter. They just need to avoid the meat and substitute servings of other protein sources, such as cooked dried beans, pulses, soya foods, peas, nuts and seeds. Make sure that most meals are accompanied by a serving of a vitamin C rich food to increase the uptake of iron from vegetarian foods. An orange, kiwi or strawberries for dessert, or a portion of broccoli or cabbage, is sufficient to increase the iron uptake from vegetable proteins by up to 100 per cent. Avoid drinking tea with your meals, as this reduces iron uptake by up to 70 per cent – stick instead to fruit teas or to hot water with a slice of lemon. If you are eating some yoghurt or a little cheese daily, in addition to a varied whole food diet, your calcium intake should be sufficient and any leafy green vegetable and nuts and seeds will also balance out the calcium with magnesium. Vitamin D may be poorly represented in the diet if you do not eat fish and, if this is the case, see the comments below.

Balancing Vegan Needs

Vegans need to watch their diets even more closely to ensure that they are not subject to deficiencies, particularly during pregnancy. When choosing protein foods they are best served by combining grains and legumes at meals, to ensure that they get all the eight amino acids that high quality proteins deliver (see **Protein Foods**, page 58, for a brief explanation of amino acids).

A healthy vegan diet needs to include, on a daily basis, the following:

- 7 servings of vegetables
- 6–11 servings of whole grains
- 4 servings of cooked dried beans, peas, pulses, nuts, seeds or soya
- 3 servings of fruit
- 4 servings of calcium-rich foods (see page 73)
- a source of vitamin B12 (see below)

A large amount of these foods needs to be eaten, to make up for any potential short-fall of iron, zinc and B6 which would come from meat consumption. A diet very high in grains and vegetables is also high in phytates (from grains) and oxylates (from dark green leafy vegetables), which can interfere with the uptake of these minerals, so more is needed (and remember the advice about vitamin C rich foods and tea in relation to iron given previously). Fish and dairy are our main sources of dietary vitamin D, which works with calcium and magnesium to grow healthy bones. The other source of vitamin D is sunlight, which allows our skin to manufacture this vitamin. As they don't eat fish and dairy products, vegans are well advised to make sure that they get sufficient sun exposure (but obviously not so much as to burn). A good quality, pregnancy-formulated supplement which gives 400 ius of vitamin D is advisable.

The supplement should also contain 50 mcg of vitamin B12, as this is the nutrient most likely to be deficient in a vegan diet. Sources of vitamin B12 are all of animal origin, or come from bacterial contamination or yeast fermentation. It is suspected that the reason why strictly vegan communities in some Eastern countries do not suffer from vitamin B12 deficiencies is that they unwittingly eat foods which are contaminated with bacteria, yeasts or even insects, and this is sufficient to provide for their B12 needs. It is generally accepted that purely plant sources of B12, for instance from spirulina, cannot be absorbed by humans and so vegans need to get their B12 from yeasts. Brewer's yeast and wheatgerm are valuable add-ins to the vegan diet, as are fermented soya products such as miso and tempeh. Seaweeds are also powerhouses of nutrients, such as iodine, iron and magnesium, both for vegans and non-vegans alike.

It is important for vegans, as with all mothers, to follow a careful eating plan throughout breast-feeding, as well as during pregnancy. On average, babies of vegan mothers tend to be smaller than other babies and their nutrient needs must be attended to. A vegan mother, unless she supplements with vitamin B12, is likely to pass less of this vitamin to her baby. Vitamin B12 deficient babies are at higher risk of developing nerve damage, anaemia and other deficiency disorders.

EATING PLANS

Let's have a look at some eating plans from pregnant women who were interested in optimising their diets, and review suggestions about how to make adaptations to their diets for the better.

Jane's Food Diary

Score: ✓✓✓✓

Breakfast
soya yoghurt with kiwi and strawberries and pumpkin seeds
wholemeal toast, scrape of butter and 100 per cent fruit jam
cup of tea

Snack
3 tbsp cottage cheese with grapes
camomile tea

Lunch
large baked potato
hummus
large mixed salad with avocado, sunflower seeds and lean
     bacon bits
orange
water
fruit tea

Snack
mixed grain Ryvita with tahini and tomato slices
fennel tea

Evening meal
salmon
cauliflower in a parsley sauce
julienne carrots with grated ginger
baked sweet potatoes
leafy side salad
stewed fruit with Greek yoghurt
mint tea

Evening snack
pear
camomile tea

Jane's food plan is ideal for pregnancy. She manages to get a good variety of foods into her day and eats plenty of vitamin, mineral and fibre rich foods as well as drinking sufficient hydrating liquids. Her intake of essential fats comes from the fresh pumpkin seeds, sunflower seeds and hummus (sesame seed paste is an ingredient). She eats plenty of whole grains and foods that are rich in iron, zinc and calcium, as well as managing to get in a portion of yellow/orange fruit/vegetables and dark green leafy vegetables. If all of Jane's eating plans follow this one, she and her baby should be doing well.

Jasmin's Food Diary

Score: ✓✓✓

Breakfast
2 hard boiled eggs
2 slices of brown toast with butter
1 small glass of orange juice
2 cups of Earl Grey tea with milk and honey

Snack
muesli bar

Lunch
steamed fillet white fish
mixed green salad with mayonnaise
bean salad
water
cup of tea with honey

Snack
apple
2 cups of fruit tea

Evening meal
chicken breast (no skin)
new potatoes
broccoli
carrots
fruit salad with almond biscuit and scoop of ice cream
water

Snack

slice of brown toast with almond nut butter
camomile tea with honey

Jasmin has a pretty good diet and is successful at making sure that she gets enough fruit and vegetables, but her calcium intake is a third too low and she is also getting too little vitamin D. Her iron and zinc levels are quite good. As she is avoiding red meat she is reducing the saturated fat content of the diet. She could substitute whole grains for the refined grains (wholemeal toast instead of brown toast for breakfast and oatcakes instead of toast for her late snack). She relies on sugary foods to boost her energy levels (the muesli bar, almond biscuits, ice cream and honey), as well as looking for a caffeine lift from her tea (even though she only drinks three cups, it is best if she does not go beyond this). She would be better off substituting a bowl of sugar-free muesli with sliced fruit and milk or rye crackers or oatcakes with a topping as snacks. If she made a point of eating plain yoghurt as snacks or for dessert this would also give her more calcium. If she ate more whole grains, and made the suggested substitutions, her energy levels would probably last for longer.

Jasmin also does not get enough omega-3 fats. A better option would be to make a salad dressing with flax or walnut oil instead of using mayonnaise, which is high in hydrogenated and saturated fats, and to substitute an oily fish, such as salmon or sardines, for the white fish, which would also give her more vitamin D.

Carina's Food Diary
. . . .
Score: ✓ ✓

Breakfast
Shreddies with semi-skimmed milk
½ plain bagel with marmalade
a glass of grapefruit juice
prenatal vitamin

Snack
2 plain biscuits
decaffeinated tea with milk

Lunch
chicken and sweetcorn baguette
low fat fruit yoghurt
diet coke

Snack
apple

Evening meal
pasta shells with bottled tomato pasta sauce and Cheddar
1 piece garlic bread
reduced fat chocolate mousse
mineral water

Snack
hot chocolate

Carina's diet is fairly unvaried, depending quite heavily on
refined wheat products. There are not enough fruit and vegeta-

bles in her eating plan. Her dependence on low vitality foods with few nutrients (the diet coke, white baguette and garlic bread, chocolate mousse and hot chocolate powder) means that she is not getting the best out of her diet for both her sake and the baby's. She needs to replace these with vegetable juices, whole grains and plain yoghurts. Carina also needs to replace some of her brown bread with whole grains and to base more meals around eggs, fish, pulses or tofu. Relying on packaged foods also means that she is getting too much salt.

She does not drink enough hydrating liquids and it would be best if she could make a point of drinking more fruit teas, water and diluted fresh juices. She is taking a prenatal supplement, which is a good thing, particularly as she is low in folic acid and vitamin D, but she could be getting a lot more from her diet.

Sally's Food Diary

Score: ✓ ✓ ✓ ✓

Breakfast
grapefruit
scrambled egg on wholemeal toast
blackcurrant tea

Snack
oatcake with almond nut butter
fruit tea

Lunch
cottage cheese with freshly cut spring onions
toasted pumpernickel bread with tahini

large green leafy salad with yellow peppers, tomatoes, black
olives and steamed baby potatoes and French dressing
water

Snack
sharon fruit
ginger and lemon tea

Evening meal
lentil soup
stir-fry (tofu, onion, mangetout, carrots, water-chestnuts,
cabbage) with brown rice
frozen banana with mild live yoghurt and ground pumpkin
seeds
peppermint tea

Other
water throughout the day

Sally is a vegetarian and manages to balance her diet well to the
benefit of her and her baby. She manages to eat mineral and
vitamin rich foods and to have a variety of foods in her plan. She
is conscious of good sources of essential fats and manages to get
sufficient protein without depending too heavily on one source.
Her calcium and magnesium levels are excellent. While the ratio
of fats to proteins and carbohydrates is on the high side, Sally
does not have a weight problem and most of her fats are from
sources that are rich in the healthy mono- and poly-unsaturated
fats. While her calcium, and other nutrient levels are excellent,
she is low in vitamin D, as is typical of many vegetarians, so she
may need to supplement this.

Annette's Food Diary

Score: ✓

Breakfast
cornflakes with semi-skimmed milk and sprinkle-on artificial
    sweetener
banana
hot water with lemon

Snack
½ flapjack
fresh orange juice
iron supplement

Lunch
cream of mushroom soup (tinned)
crackers and cheese
2 tangerines
mineral water

Snack
yoghurt coated raisins
fruit tea

Evening meal
ricotta ravioli with tomato sauce
fruit fromage frais

Other
water throughout the day

Annette makes little attempt to vary her diet away from wheat and dairy based foods. She is a vegetarian, and because she does not manage it very well, she does not get enough protein or calories to meet the needs of a growing baby. Her diet is also low in essential fats, vitamins A, B3, folic acid and D, as well as the minerals iron and zinc. Her salt intake is more than 50 per cent too high. Although she takes an iron supplement with orange juice to increase the absorption rate, she could get more iron (as well as many other minerals) from her diet by just adding in a portion of leafy green vegetables, a portion of beans or pulses and some seeds, and having a small glass of orange juice alongside these. She would be better off taking a multi-formula prenatal supplement to get a good balance of nutrients and to make up for the deficiencies in her diet.

Annette needs to eat a more substantial lunch and to concentrate on eating healthier snacks. Whole grain breakfast cereals, fresh soups and vegetarian protein substitutes would be other improvements. Finally, I don't believe that using artificial sweeteners when pregnant is a good idea. Research has shown that they are linked to neurological damage in rats, and I would not advise using them during pregnancy.

Vanessa's Food Diary

Score: ✓ ✓

Breakfast
bran muffin (shop bought)
banana
cup of tea

Snack
packet of pretzels
orange

Lunch
vegetable sushi and marinated tofu pieces
pre-prepared fresh fruit salad
water

Snack
packet of nuts and dried fruit
cup of tea

Evening meal
carton of fresh minestrone soup
seafood pizza
green salad with low-cal vinaigrette
low fat fruit yoghurt
clementine

Vanessa is working hard throughout her pregnancy and relies heavily on takeaway foods, as a result her diet is low in several nutrients, including B vitamins, vitamin A, iron and zinc. Despite the fact that she relies on pre-prepared foods, she is health conscious and chooses 'freshly made' ones and so her salt levels are reasonable. The calorie count for this day is too low, but this may simply be an accident of this menu. Other easy options for a takeaway lunch could include jacket potatoes with tuna, coleslaw or beans, a flask of fresh soup, a falafel stuffed pitta pocket or a portion of chicken with salad. She also does not get enough dark green and yellow vegetables and could incorporate pre-cut vegetables with a dip at lunchtime. Vanessa is not a vegetarian, so in view of her low iron and zinc levels she should include a little red meat from time to time. By eating more oily fish and including some seeds as snacks she could also improve her intake of essential fats.

CAUTIONARY FOOD TALES

Some foods are best avoided when pregnant as they can have a detrimental impact on the baby. They may, for example, harbour bacteria, which can result in problems for the foetus. This can cause a lot of anxiety if a mother-to-be finds she is pregnant and knows she has eaten, say, some soft cheese the day before. It is important to get this into proportion. There is a 1 in 29,000 risk of listeria in pregnancy, which is considerably less than the risk of getting hit by a car (1 in 6,000). Other countries take a much more relaxed attitude. In France, for instance, they carry on quite happily eating soft cheeses and paté throughout pregnancy. On the other hand, I have met a couple whose child's life was devastated when the mother contracted food poisoning at a party and their baby ended up being severely handicapped. The message here is to not panic if you have eaten any foods which are cautioned against, but to be cautious in future. Here are the foods to avoid, or prepare correctly, and the reasons why:

prepare salads and vegetables properly

Fresh vegetables and salads, whether bought ready prepared from the supermarket or home grown, need to be washed thoroughly to remove any possible traces of soil which could be contaminated with bacteria, including toxoplasmosis. Avoid potatoes which have sprouted or which have green patches, as these will contain a highly toxic compound called solanine.

prepare meat properly

Most cases of toxoplasmosis are contracted through people eating contaminated meat. One third of all chickens are infected with salmonella, and meat is another potential source of salmonella (see eggs below). Antibiotic resistant salmonella found in fast foods, such as hamburgers and other take-away meat dishes, has recently created an epidemic of illness. Meat and poultry must be defrosted thoroughly before cooking, and cooked sufficiently so that the internal temperature of the meat is 54 degrees C/140 degrees F – or until the juices run clear when you test the meat with a skewer. Wash your hands before and after handling meat, and do not use the same chopping board for uncooked meat as you do for fruit, vegetables or bread, or indeed anything which may be eaten without cooking (it is best to keep two distinctly different chopping boards for these two purposes). Wash knives thoroughly after cutting raw meat and before using them for other purposes. Store all raw or defrosting meat or poultry on the lowest shelf in your refrigerator to avoid any contamination of other foods by dripping liquids. Store cooked and uncooked food well away from each other, and cover food properly. Meats normally eaten raw, such as cured Parma ham, should also be considered suspect.

avoid soft and blue cheeses
Soft cheeses and blue cheeses, including Camembert, Brie, Vignotte, Stilton, Cambozola, Danish blue, Dolcelatte, Roquefort, goat's and sheep's (ewe's) cheeses, can harbour high levels of listeria. Listeriosis can lead to flu-like symptoms which, even at mild levels, can lead to miscarriage, stillbirth or severe illness in a newborn baby. Hard pasteurised cheeses such as Cheddar can still be enjoyed as can cottage cheese, though unpasteurised cheeses such as Parmesan may be best avoided.

eat liver only in moderation and not at all during the first 12 weeks
Standard advice for pregnant women is to avoid liver due to its high vitamin A content. However, only one recorded case has

been noted of this affecting a baby and the mother was eating liver daily throughout her pregnancy. USA nutritionist Elizabeth Somer has broken ranks by saying that moderate intake is not only safe but also nutritious, and I agree with her. Limit liver during pregnancy to a small portion (85 g/3 oz) once every three weeks. At 36,000 ius per 85-g/3-oz portion this would be equivalent to 1,700 ius per day of vitamin A, which is acceptable, though to be on the safe side do not eat liver products in the first 12 weeks of your pregnancy. If you eat liver regularly (a small portion once every three weeks) you need to avoid any supplements with vitamin A in them, and choose those based on beta-carotene instead. Liver is such a rich source of nutrients, including iron, zinc, B vitamins and folic acid, that it is almost the ideal nutritional supplement to make up for deficiencies, but caution must be exercised. It is also probably a good idea to make sure that the liver you eat is organic, because the liver is the organ of detoxification for all animals, and this means that if you do not eat organic liver you can potentially ingest the harmful chemicals the animal may be harbouring in its liver. Best of all, eat calves' liver, which has probably not had a chance to be overly contaminated.

eggs, poultry and raw egg based foods
Salmonella is the most common form of food poisoning and symptoms include sickness, diarrhoea and fever. To avoid problems make sure any poultry is properly cooked (see above) and ensure that eggs are cooked so that both the white and yellow parts are solid. Discard any cracked eggs, and do not allow any raw egg to come into contact with other foods. Avoid foods which might contain raw egg, such as fresh mayonnaise, home-made ice cream and chocolate mousse.

paté, ready-to-eat poultry and cook-chill foods

These are other foods which have been found to be risky as they can contain listeria. Heat pre-cooked ready meals until they are piping hot to kill off any bacteria. The worst offenders, in recent tests, turned out to be chilled cooked chicken, which harboured high levels of listeria and salmonella. Paté which is canned or shrink wrapped and marked pasteurised is OK from the point of view of food poisoning risk, though I am not crazy about shrink wrapped plastic on anything (see **The Womb: A Pollution Free Zone**, page 17).

unpasteurised milks

Unpasteurised milk can be a breeding ground for a number of different bacteria. Make sure that any milk you drink is pasteurised, sterilised or UHT (ultra heat treated). If you normally drink goat's or ewe's milk, make sure that they are also treated, as it is possible for unpasteurised goat's or ewe's milk to harbour toxoplasmosis. Also avoid soft-whip ice cream from ice cream machines and vans.

peanuts (monkeynuts, groundnuts)

These are not really nuts at all, but are a member of the legume family. This makes sense when you think about how peanuts come lined up in pods in the same way as other beans. They are also called groundnuts because the runners grow under the ground. While peanuts are an excellent source of proteins and unsaturated fats, they are also high in compounds called lectins to which some people are highly allergic. There has been a sharp increase in the number of children who have developed life-threatening, anaphylactic responses to peanuts. It is thought that this is because of the increased use of the peanut, which is a cheap ingredient, in a wide variety of convenience foods such as biscuits and other savoury and sweet prepared meals and snacks, and it is possible that babies may be sensitised while still in the womb. Peanuts are often contaminated with aflatoxins and so if you do choose to eat peanuts avoid those that are stale. It is probably wise, during pregnancy, to avoid peanut based foods to reduce the risk of allergy in your child if you belong to a family with allergies, such as asthma, hay fever, eczema or psoriasis, or have known food allergies. The second most common and dangerous allergy, after peanuts, is to sesame seeds. Unless you have a specific allergy, real nuts, such as almonds or walnuts, and seeds other than sesame, such as sunflower or pumpkin, are much less likely to be a problem and are highly nutritious.

shellfish and raw fish

As there is a fairly high risk of food poisoning from shellfish, particularly raw shellfish, you may be happier avoiding them altogether. If you do eat them, make sure that they are totally fresh and come from a reliable supplier. Raw fish, such as in sushi, may be a source of parasites.

WEIGHT DURING PREGNANCY

The average woman (have you ever met this person?) needs around 2,000 calories per day, but while she is pregnant she needs an additional 200 calories in the last trimester, and while she is breast-feeding she needs an additional 500 calories. 'Eating for two' is no longer seriously recommended, but you will probably find that your appetite naturally increases to accommodate these needs.

During pregnancy a woman of average build and height will gain between 11.5–16 kg/25–35 lb, and the average weight gain is 12.5 kg/28 lb. Most of this consists of the baby and its 'support services' (see box below), but some is likely to be increased body weight, which will need to be shed afterwards (a process that is helped by breast-feeding). Extra fat is built up by the body during pregnancy to provide energy reserves for breast-feeding, so take advantage of this to help get back into shape (see **Breast-feeding**, page 183). If you gain much more than 16 kg/35 lb you may find the extra weight hard to lose afterwards. A good way of assessing if you are putting on too much weight is to measure your upper thighs every couple of weeks. Your upper thigh measurement should stay about the same throughout the pregnancy.

weight increase in pregnancy is due to:

baby	30 per cent
placenta	7 per cent
amniotic fluid	9 per cent
increase in weight of uterus and breasts	12 per cent
extra fat and fluid retention	25 per cent
increase in blood volume	17 per cent

Caution: Beware of a sudden and excessive weight gain after the 24th week as this can be a sign of pre-eclampsia.

The anguish that many women feel about their weight is often compounded when they fall pregnant. They worry on two fronts – is the weight they are putting on acceptable (not too much and not too little?), and will they be able to lose any excess weight afterwards? Ideally, your weight needs to be in the normal range for your height for six months before you conceive. If you are seriously underweight or overweight this may affect your chances of fertility or lead to complications during the pregnancy. However, if you need to lose some weight, pregnancy is not the time to go on a calorie-restricted diet. Restricting calories usually means restricting nutrients, and this can adversely affect you and the baby. On the other hand, eating a healthy, nutrient-rich diet during pregnancy may well result in the pleasant surprise, if you are overweight, of losing some body fat. If you are already heavy your body will not need to make more fat stores to nourish the developing baby, and eating healthily can lead to body weight stabilising itself.

If you are underweight, you may be advised to eat more calories during pregnancy to make up some of the weight. This is most easily achieved by eating more high-calorie and nutrient-dense foods. Make sure that you eat more fresh nuts and seeds and that any dairy produce you eat is the full fat variety. Being underweight can adversely affect the chances of conception, and is also a factor in producing low birth-weight babies. Anorexics, along with serious athletes and dancers, can find that their puberty is delayed by several years and that menstruation ceases. This is no surprise when you realise that their bodies are trying to protect them from the onslaught of pregnancy which demands a high price in terms of nutrients.

to help stabilise your weight:
- Avoid processed convenience foods and snacks.
- Snack on fresh fruit and vegetable sticks instead of on sugary, salty and fatty snacks.
- Make sure the fats in your diet come from oily fish, fresh nuts, fresh seeds, coconut, avocados and small amounts of added fats from cold-pressed olive oil, flax oil, walnut oil and sesame oil.
- Eat low fat dairy products such as skimmed milk, cottage cheese and low fat yoghurts, but avoid those with added sugar (such as some yoghurts). There is just as much calcium in low fat dairy produce as in higher fat dairy produce.
- Avoid too much butter, cheese and animal fats if you are aiming to lose weight. Avoid processed margarines and fatty foods such as pies, crisps, buns and biscuits. At the

same time eat fats that are healthy and needed for the
growth of your baby. If you are underweight make sure
that you increase the healthy fats in your diet significantly.

● Cut back on sugar and sugary foods. Instead, rely on
natural sources of sweetness, which also come packed with
vitamins and minerals, such as fruit and dried fruit. If you
absolutely have to sweeten your drinks, use a little fructose
(fruit sugar available from health food shops) or honey.

● Drink plenty of filtered water – at least eight large glasses
a day (a total of 2 litres / 3½ pints daily).

● Never skip a meal – if you deny yourself, you deny your
baby.

● Avoid blood sugar problems by snacking regularly to
maintain energy levels without resorting to energy props.
Keep a good supply of nutritious snacks, such as fresh nuts,
seeds, dips, wholemeal crackers, fruit, yoghurts or lean
cold cuts easily to hand in the refrigerator or cupboard.

● Keep nourishing snacks in your desk drawer at work, if
you do not have access to a refrigerator, such as Twiglets,
fresh nuts, oatcakes or dried fruit mix, and fresh fruit.

healthy snacks and treats

● a jar of fresh nuts in the refrigerator
● oatcakes spread with almond nut butter
● some small pots of yoghurts
● fresh soups
● packets of fresh sunflower or pumpkin seeds
● Chinese or Japanese rice crackers
● fruit cubes and strawberries dipped in dark chocolate and
kept in the refrigerator
● half a wholemeal pitta stuffed with tomato and red onion
slices
● dried fruit (mix with nuts and seeds)

- wholemeal crackers and snacks
- dips such as hummus or guacamole eaten with wholemeal pitta fingers, crackers or crudités
- fruit smoothies
- yoghurt with puréed fruit and a sprinkling of chopped walnuts
- cottage cheese with apple sauce or pear slices
- half an avocado with flaked salmon in a mild mustard/yoghurt sauce
- strips of ham or turkey wrapped around papaya chunks or 'soft' dried apricots

This advice holds true both if you need to gain weight and if you need to lose weight. A common mistake for women aiming to gain weight is to believe that the only thing they need to do is to eat more calories. What is just as important as calories is the need to eat a nutrient rich diet that gives them the basic building blocks that they and the baby need. This means eating vitamin and mineral rich foods and also ensuring that fats come from healthy sources, as they are also used as building blocks to make cell membranes, hormones and nervous tissue. If you have trouble eating enough calories at main meals, then eat several smaller meals and snacks, and aim to eat every three hours.

ORGANIC EATING

One modern day problem, which pregnant women are having to deal with for the first time in history, is the addition of a cocktail of pesticides to our food. There are several reasons why a pregnant woman, or a woman contemplating pregnancy, would want as much of her food as possible to be organic.

The first, and most fascinating reason, especially for anyone who is interested in improving her chances of fertility, is that a study has shown that organic herds of animals grew more fertile over three generations, while fertility in conventionally reared herds declined slightly.

Secondly, the nutrient levels in organic fruit and vegetables have been demonstrated in some studies to be higher when compared to non-organic produce. While not conclusive, this is persuasive. In my opinion the produce also usually tastes better.

Thirdly, it has recently come to light that vegetarian women have five times the average risk of producing boy babies with a condition called hypospadias, where the penis is not properly formed, and which usually requires corrective surgery within the first two years of life. One in 150 boys are now born with hypospadias, sometimes having genitals so similar to a girl's as to make sexing the child difficult. For the most part, hypospadias manifests itself by having the opening of the penis in the wrong place, for example half way along, because the urine tube has not closed up properly. The incidence has increased from 1 in 300 boys only a few decades ago, and it is strongly suspected that the reason for this is that the higher fruit, vegetable and grain consumption of vegetarian mothers is exposing them to more pesticides than non-vegetarian mothers.

The solution is probably to eat foods, whenever possible, which are organic and are therefore certified as not having been sprayed by these potentially dangerous chemicals. There is no question that a diet high in fruit and vegetables is one of the healthiest ways forward and that eating non-organic plant produce is better than eating no plant produce at all, so do not use this as a reason to justify not eating lots of fruit and vegetables.

Finally, and most disturbingly, compounds are finding their way into the milk of breast-feeding mothers, thus exposing babies to chemicals in their first weeks of life. This does not necessarily negate the benefits of breast-feeding, but does suggest that women need to do all they can to reduce their exposure to pesticides and other chemicals (see **Your Diet While Breast-feeding,** page 183, for more information).

It is still important to wash organic produce well. There have been recent scares about organic produce harbouring the E.coli 0157 organism though this has since been discounted. Nevertheless by preparing vegetables properly you can avoid this very small risk if it exists.

JUNK FOOD JUNKIES

As you recline on the sofa choosing which chocolate your baby would really like you to eat today and reading about what is a healthy diet for pregnancy, think for a moment about how you are actually going to make all this work.

Eating healthily isn't made easy, surrounded as we are by temptation. Sugary, salty and fatty foods are manufactured by the food giants precisely because they are so addictive. Sugary foods in particular affect blood sugar levels and brain chemicals, which makes them difficult to kick. But now is a time when you really can't afford to load up your body with empty calories from sugar, or take in loads of salt, which can affect water balance, or eat too many of the wrong kind of fats, which do not serve any purpose in building healthy nervous tissue for your baby. The majority of people do not eat the five portions of fruit and vegetables daily recommended by government health agencies. Might you be one of these people? How close is your diet to Eating for a Perfect Pregnancy? Of course, there is nothing wrong with occasional treats, but if you are filling up on crisps, biscuits, snack bars or white bread at the expense of eating fruit, vegetables and whole grains, you need to work out a way forward.

A word here, also, about sugar substitutes. You may be curbing your use of sugar with artificial sweeteners. Artificial sweeteners do nothing to curb a taste for sugary foods, and really promote it at the expense of changing habits towards healthier options. It is also true to say that the majority of commercially artificially sweetened foods are usually nutritional paupers and are best avoided. There is no convincing evidence one way or the other about the advisability of using sweeteners in pregnancy, however logic suggests that it is best to derive natural sweetness from fruit and juices. If you enjoy strong tastes you may want to experiment with blackstrap molasses which is immensely nutrient rich and is delicious, for instance, if you use a little in porridge or in baking. Another option is to use, in moderation, fructose (fruit sugar available at health food shops), as it does not have such a negative effect on blood sugar levels as sugar.

Tips for Avoiding Temptation

If you are addicted to sweet, salty and fatty foods you may already be beating yourself up with guilt about your diet being less than perfect while you are pregnant. Well stop now. It will not do any good at all to compound your negative feeling by berating yourself and feeling miserable. The only possible way forward is to take each little victory at a time, concentrate on being nice to yourself, and reward yourself when you eat healthily for yourself and your baby by doing other non-food related things you enjoy.

Here are some ways to help you make sure you eat as well as you are able for these vital and exciting nine months.

● Be prepared. If you know you are venturing into the jaws of temptation, say tea at a friend's house, take something with you that you can eat instead of the proffered cake and biscuits – such as some nuts, fruit or bran muffins, or a home baked cake, or one bought from a good quality bakery, made using wholemeal flour, banana or dried fruit and butter or olive oil, instead of white flour, sugar and margarine.

- Don't skip breakfast, and make sure that you eat regularly. If you base these meals, and any snacks in between, on wholesome nutritious foods you are less likely to suffer from cravings.

- If you feel a really strong urge for less than terrific food, make a deal with yourself. Tell yourself you can have some of the food, but only after you have had a healthy snack and a large glass of water or fruit tea (see page 109 for suggestions of snacks). If you still feel like the splurge after that, go ahead, but be moderate. At least you will have given your body some nutrients to work alongside the doughnut or cream cake.

- Stock up the cupboards with lots of delicious and tempting foods you enjoy which will also nurture you and your baby. Don't get caught short!

- Eating during pregnancy is not about denial or deprivation. Actually healthy eating is never about these sentiments. If these are the emotions you feel when turning down your particular nemesis, then these are psychological messages that need working on and not physical ones. Give yourself treats, and plenty of them. Just work out which ones you will enjoy and which will still nurture you and your baby.

- Out of sight is often out of mind. Ask your family to join with you in your Eating for a Perfect Pregnancy and to keep temptation out of your way. Your whole family's health will benefit as a result.

- Eating meals and snacks which balance proteins with wholegrain carbohydrates is the best way to de-programme yourself from craving sweet foods. This means eating, for instance, cooked buckwheat pasta twists mixed in with a salad containing strips of ham or hard boiled egg instead of pasta with a vegetable sauce or a jacket potato filled with tuna salad instead of the same jacket potato with just butter.

● Eliminating coffee and alcohol, apart from being best for your baby, will also reduce the degree of blood sugar swings you experience and so should help to reduce cravings for sweet foods. Of course, you may be tempted to substitute the 'lift' you get from your morning coffee with something sweet instead, but if you can avoid this pitfall, by eating a protein and complex carbohydrate based meal, you will be able to manage your cravings better.

● One of the best ways to get rid of the need for a pudding after a meal, which all too often is just that little too much, and in addition is laden with unnecessary sugar, is to eat a piece of juicy and delicious fruit and then to follow that swiftly by cleaning your teeth. The fruit gives just enough sugar to get rid of the craving, and brushing your teeth makes your mouth feel clean so it becomes less appealing to sully it with something sticky and sweet.

ELIMINATION DIETS

Elimination diets are those which avoid particular foods, or food groups. It is usually not a good idea to start an elimination diet once you know you are pregnant because while you might feel better, the metabolic shifts that happen when you eliminate foods to which you are sensitive can include detoxification of chemicals stored in fat tissues, and there is always a chance that this will adversely affect the baby. It is perfectly safe, however, to eliminate a particular food (as long as you make sensible substitutions). And in case you love sugar and sugary foods, I'm sorry to tell you that these are not a food group and can quite happily be eliminated! The food groups were outlined at the beginning of this chapter and as long as you choose from within each group then your diet will be balanced and healthy for you and your baby.

If you have been following a regime before pregnancy which avoids particular foods that do not agree with you, say wheat products or milk, it is fine to continue with this as long as you choose good alternatives. This is true of any foods in any group. If, for instance, oranges or bananas don't agree with you, eat some fruit that does, such as plums or cantaloupe melons. If you don't like red meat, eat poultry, fish or legumes. If wheat makes you bloat, eat brown rice, buckwheat or potatoes. Calcium rich options have already been given if you dislike milk (or it dislikes you). Just refer back to the relevant sections in **The Food Pyramid**, page 50, for other foods you can eat within each group.

GESTATIONAL DIABETES

Two or three women in a hundred, who are pregnant, develop gestational diabetes, making it a fairly common phenomenon. Gestational diabetes occurs during pregnancy, usually in the second half, and then disappears after the birth. Women who have gestational diabetes are, however, more at risk of developing diabetes later in life. It is probably the stress of the pregnancy on the pancreas, and the interaction between the hormones, that causes the condition. It is also possible that in many cases the women are 'borderline' disabetics who would have gone on to develop the condition later on. If a woman is an undiagnosed diabetic, however, she is likely to continue as a diabetic after the pregnancy. As with late-onset diabetes (diabetes which develops in adulthood rather than in childhood), the condition in pregnancy can be controlled with diet, and this is even more effective if dietary steps are instigated before, or early on, in the pregnancy. During the pregnancy the woman's urine will routinely be tested for sugar, which can signal that gestational diabetes is a problem. Some complications are more likely to be seen in a baby of a mother with gestational diabetes. Diabetic women often deliver larger babies, which can make the birth more difficult and increase the risk of a Caesarean section. The baby also has a greater risk of having hypoglycaemia (low blood sugar), of being jaundiced and of having respiratory distress problems.

Eating for a Perfect Pregnancy takes into account all of the needs of the woman with gestational diabetes, but it is worth pointing out that, if you have high sugar levels in your urine on a few consecutive tests, eating to balance blood sugar levels may be able to correct the problem. The bottom line, however, is that if you are diagnosed with this condition you need to stick more closely to the recommendations, and cheat less often. The important points to remember are:

- Make sure that all your carbohydrates are complex. Instead of sugary foods and white bread or pasta, eat bread, cakes, biscuits and pasta made from wholemeal flour or from other wholegrains.
- Avoid all sources of sugar, honey and refined carbohydrates.
- Eat a little protein with each meal — so even if you are having a complex carbohydrate for a snack, such as a rye cracker, make sure that you have, for example, a little chopped hard boiled egg, bean salad or a yoghurt alongside it.
- Make sure that you get 20–35 g of fibre daily. Fibre helps to regulate the effect that carbohydrates have on blood

sugar levels, by slowing down their release into the blood-stream. If you are not reaching your target, add up to two teaspoons of psyllium husks to your programme (see page 140).

● Eat chromium and magnesium rich foods. These two minerals are closely involved in regulating blood sugar levels. For chromium and magnesium rich foods see pages 88 and 74.

● Take a good quality pregnancy-formulated daily multivitamin that contains at least 25 mg of vitamin B3, and take up to 200 mcg of chromium per day.

CHAPTER FOUR

The Natural Remedy Cupboard

During pregnancy it is important to avoid most medicines, which can leave you wondering what to do if you have trouble sleeping or need to get your bowels moving. But in addition to medicines being off limits, many herbs are as well, so this chapter looks at herbs and therapeutic foods that are safe to take during pregnancy and which you can keep handy to deal with minor health problems.

We use herbs, and spices, every day to add flavour to cooking and as ingredients in delicious teas and drinks. Herbs also contain many vitamins, minerals and other nutrients, making them valuable additions to a varied diet. The best way to benefit from the healing powers of culinary herbs is to incorporate them liberally in your daily salads and cooking. Mostly culinary herbs are fine during pregnancy, and the quantities used in preparing foods are usually too small to have a 'pharmacological' effect. However, some very familiar culinary herbs and spices – parsley, sage and nutmeg, for example – can have an adverse effect during pregnancy if used in even low therapeutic doses.

Herbs have been used for at least a couple of thousand years as potent healers and medicines. There are many different herbs used in cultures across the world and the methods and herbs used by Chinese, Native American and European herbalists are often very different. Because herbs have such active effects, they can, in many cases, be as powerful as drugs, so using them during pregnancy needs to be done with caution, if at all.

The majority of herbs need to be avoided during pregnancy unless they are specifically prescribed by a knowledgeable practitioner. Others, however, are known to be safe during pregnancy, and have been tried and tested over time. Of course, there is always the possibility of individual reactions and if any of the 'safe' herbs give any undesirable effects, you need to be alert to this and stop them immediately. If you are adding any herbs into your regime during pregnancy, you need to do this slowly and carefully to be aware of any problems such as individual allergic reactions. It is always desirable to seek professional advice from a herbalist about using herbal remedies. It is also a good idea to make sure that any herbs you buy are from a reputable supplier. If you are gathering wild herbs, make sure that you identify the plants correctly. Follow the manufacturer's dosage guidelines carefully, and by no means fall in to the trap of thinking that 'if a little is good, then more is better' – this simply is not so, and can be dangerous.

Because an exhaustive list of herbs would be too extensive to appear here, unless a herb is listed below as 'safe' to use during pregnancy you must consider it to be unsuitable, except where you get specific advice from a suitably qualified professional – and even then still be cautious. Be wary, too, of multi-nutrient supplements which may contain herbs alongside the other ingredients – check the labels carefully.

some of the negative effects that herbs can have on a pregnancy include:

- Herbs with strong alkaloids, or volatile oils, can affect the developing baby's nervous system in the first trimester.
- Herbs that can be useful for increasing blood supply to the uterus in late pregnancy, can be potent enough to stimulate premature contractions if taken too early in the pregnancy.
- Some herbs may be able to cause liver damage to a foetus,

the main suspects being comfrey, coltsfoot and borage. (External use of comfrey as a poultice for healing wounds is still safe.)

● Herbs which increase peristalsis (the moving action) of the gut may also promote uterine contractions. If you are constipated see the advice about fibre on page 140 to promote healthy bowel movements.

● Herbs which are known to affect hormone balance and those which are used to bring on menstruation must be avoided during pregnancy. Foods which affect hormones, such as tofu, wholewheat, rye and chickpeas are fine to eat in normal quantities during pregnancy.

● Herbs which are used as de-worming compounds must be avoided in pregnancy.

● European herbal practice advises against the use of herbs such as Dong Quai during pregnancy, yet in China it is given as a blood tonic for pregnant women. You need to exercise great caution when you come across these discrepancies.

A–Z OF PREGNANCY HERBALS

Here is an alphabetical list of the herbs, and some foods, which are generally considered safe to take during pregnancy, along with their main uses for promoting a healthy pregnancy:

alfalfa Alfalfa is rich in chlorophyll (the green colouring of plants), carotenes, as well as iron, and is ideal to use as a tonic once or twice a week to help prevent **anaemia**. It is also rich in many other vitamins and minerals which support overall health.

burdock root You can use this as a dried herb from the root, or use the root itself (gobo) in cooking instead of carrots. It helps to stabilise **blood sugar levels**, supports the liver and urinary tract, and tones the uterus. Because it stimulates the liver and pancreas it helps **digestion** and is very mildly **laxative**. It can also help if you suffer from **itchy skin**.

camomile This multi-purpose herb is relaxing and helps to promote **sleep** and reduce **mental tension** and **headaches**. It is helpful for **digestion, nausea** and **heartburn**. Camomile can also be useful in reducing **cramps, constipation** and **urinary tract infections**. Make by steeping it for 10 minutes in a cup covered with a saucer to stop the useful compounds evaporating with the water. Drink up to four cups daily. (Whilst rare, some people with an allergy to ragweed may react badly to camomile. If you have a history of miscarriage or spotting within the first four months of pregnancy do not exceed one cup of camomile daily as it can help to promote menstruation.)

cherries These are rich in a **pain killing** compound and 20 cherries are equivalent to one aspirin.

cornsilk These are the silky strands between the head of sweetcorn and its covering leaves, which you infuse in boiling water. It is a mild diuretic that is useful for **water retention** and **cystitis** in pregnancy.

dandelion root and leaves Dandelion can help to promote **iron levels** in the blood. It is also a useful **digestive tonic**, and in addition helps to regulate **blood sugar levels** and **blood pressure**. In early pregnancy it can help to relieve **nausea**, and later on can reduce **itchy skin** problems. Use young dandelion leaves on salads and the dried root to make an infusion.

false unicorn This is a very bitter tasting herb, but it has strong therapeutic properties in strengthening the uterus and is particularly suited for women with a **history of**

miscarriage. Use it in tincture form (20 drops three times daily) in early pregnancy and then periodically throughout the rest of the pregnancy.

fennel Make fennel tea or juice the bulb for **morning sickness**, **indigestion** or **gas**.

garlic This bulb has many properties, including improving blood flow and acting as a **blood purifier**. Garlic can help to reduce the risk of **pre-eclampsia**, and has **antiseptic**, **antibacterial** and **antiviral** properties. Ideally include one clove daily in your food.

ginger One of the most useful **digestive aids** and **anti-nausea** remedies. Grate a little into a cup and steep in boiling water for 10 minutes before drinking. You may wish to add a little honey. Do not use a strong concoction more than a couple of times a day (which is perfectly safe), as large doses can stimulate blood flow to the pelvis to help bring on periods. Avoid ginger if you have gastric or peptic ulcers. The ginger and fennel drink on page 150 is sufficiently diluted to be safe to use.

green tea This tea contains powerful antioxidants and has less than 25 per cent of the caffeine of normal tea. You can use it to **bathe insect bites**, or to soothe **inflammation** and even **sunburn** (though staying in the shade in strong sun is even better). Make the tea as usual, allow it to cool, then apply with cotton wool.

kelp This is a sea vegetable which, along with all seaweeds, is a rich source of iodine, chlorophyll and many of the trace minerals. It is useful as a **general tonic** throughout pregnancy and can support the **thyroid function** of the developing baby. You can add chopped kelp/kombu leaves to soups, or grate dried kelp in a grinder on to savoury foods.

lavender You can add a pinch of lavender to other teas such as camomile. It is soothing, helps lift **depression** and reduces **anxiety**. It is also useful to relieve **gas** and **indigestion**. Best of all, you can add a handful of lavender to a warm bath to soak in.

lemon A lemon squeezed into hot water is the traditional remedy for soothing **sore throats** and **catarrh**, and a little honey helps it to slip down even more easily.

lemon balm This herb is great for reducing **tension** and for promoting **digestion**. Use about a tablespoon of the dried herb and steep in a covered cup for 15 minutes. It is ideal to combine with camomile and lavender tea.

lime flower Flowers of the lime, or linden tree, are helpful for **headaches, nasal secretions** and **sinus discomfort**. They are also useful for **high blood pressure, sleeping problems, anxiety** and **tension**. Drink no more than three cups a day. (High blood pressure must always be checked by your doctor.)

meadowsweet This herb contains a pain relieving substance, salicylic acid, which is related to aspirin, but which is more gentle as it comes with other factors. Helps to relieve **pain, inflammation** and eases the **digestive tract, heartburn** and **diarrhoea**. Drink a maximum of two cups daily.

mint Made into a tea this is a powerful **digestive aid**, and can help to steady **morning sickness**. Use it regularly after meals if your stomach tends to be unsettled.

nettle This common weed is a powerful blood supporter and helps to counteract **anaemia** if taken regularly throughout pregnancy. It is rich in many vitamins and minerals and helps to support kidney health, reduce **varicose veins** and decrease the likelihood of **haemorrhage** at the birth. Steep a handful of nettle leaves (wear protective gloves!) in a litre/1¾ pints of boiling water for one hour. A more convenient option is to buy freeze-dried nettle capsules.

oats Porridge late at night can help ensure a good night's **sleep** by balancing blood sugar levels and raising serotonin levels in the brain.

oatstraw Oatstraw tea helps to promote relaxed **nerves** as well as improving muscle function, reducing **cramps** and preventing **insomnia**.

oregano Add it to food to help to reduce **gas** problems.

partridgeberry This herb is an ideal **uterine tonic**, as well as a tonic for the **nervous system**. Steep the herb to make a tea and also combine it with other teas.

red raspberry leaves While more commonly used towards the end of pregnancy, raspberry leaves are safe to take as a tea throughout pregnancy to help **tone up the uterus**, due to its active compound, frangarine. It is also rich in iron. It is used to reduce the risk of **haemorrhage** at birth.

rose hips Rose hips are particularly rich in vitamin C, which supports the **immune system**, improves **connective tissue**, helps with **bone building** and is used for **energy**. They are most useful if used throughout the pregnancy.

tarragon This herb can help reduce **gas** and **flatulence**.

wild yam Traditionally wild yam is used to help **prevent miscarriages**. It can also help reduce **nausea**, **cramping**, **muscular tension** and **intestinal gas**, and in addition is a **liver strengthener**. It is best used as a tincture, 15 drops two or three times a day. Use 30 drops every 4 hours for more serious problems such as **hyperemesis** (extreme vomiting as a result of **morning sickness**) or a threatened miscarriage (always consult your doctor for both of these conditions).

yellow dock This is another herb that can help ward off **anaemia** as it is rich in iron and stimulates the liver.

Apart from making teas and poultices to ease what ails you, you can adopt a preventive approach by making nutrient rich juices and nourishing smoothies. Of course, you can eat a carrot or apple, for instance, but if you make a juice with three carrots and two apples you are getting a super-charge of nutrients. Juices should not be used as a substitute for eating proper meals, but they are an excellent way of taking concentrated and highly absorbable sources of nutrients. If you make smoothies you can add a number of nutrient rich ingredients to the basic formula (which may consist of milk, soya milk or live yoghurt with added soft fruit), such as wheatgerm for B-vitamins, spirulina for iron and magnesium, nut butters for essential fats or brewer's yeast for B-vitamins and chromium, or try adding a little Manuka (New Zealand) honey for its antiseptic properties, but also because it tastes good!

Part Three

THE TRIMESTERS

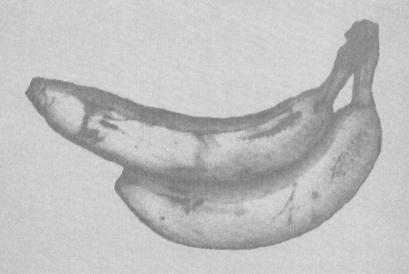

CHAPTER FIVE

The First Trimester

You are pregnant! Congratulations!

This may be your first pregnancy in which case, if you are like me, you will be reading every scrap of information you can lay your hands on. A part of you may be becoming more and more engrossed in the excitement of it all, and yet another part may be half scaring yourself to death with what you read. One friend of mine, when given a couple of pregnancy manuals, happily chucked them to one side proclaiming 'Ignorance is bliss, I shall just let Mother Nature and the doctors get on with it'. Well maybe she was right, but I happen to know that she had a pretty good diet and 'clean' lifestyle – and of course she produced a happy and healthy baby. What works for some women doesn't for others, and vice versa.

This could be a second, or later, pregnancy for you. While second-time-around parents are usually more relaxed about pregnancy and child-rearing (they've been there before!), you may be becoming more aware of the impact that diet can have, or you may be interested in avoiding complications you experienced previously.

A perfect example of the way nutrition can help second time around is the case of a lady I know who, the first time (when she was 38) took a year to become pregnant. She was diagnosed with fibroids (benign lumps in the womb) and endometriosis (tissue from the womb which attaches to other parts of the body), conditions that affect 80 per cent and 10 per cent of women of reproductive age respectively and are linked to reduced fertility or infertility. When she finally conceived she experienced strong sugar cravings, put on quite a lot of weight and had terrible heartburn throughout her pregnancy. After this experience she became fascinated with what nutrition might be able to do for her, adjusted her diet to that of Eating for a Perfect Pregnancy and took her pre-conceptual supplements. The change was remarkable. She did not want to delay for long in trying for another baby, as she felt she was 'getting on' in reproductive terms, and so was delighted when she conceived her second, and after that her third, child within one month of deciding to try for a baby. She also had no discomfort or complications during the next two pregnancies and has all the energy, in her early forties, needed to deal with three children under the age of four.

WHAT IS HAPPENING TO YOU AND YOUR BABY

week 3 The baby's entire genetic make-up was decided at that magical moment of conception. Because pregnancy is always calculated from the first day of the last period, on the day of conception you are already technically two weeks pregnant!

week 4 You may still be unaware that you are pregnant, though you can do a urine pregnancy test that looks for raised levels of hCG hormone (human chorionic gonadotrophin) from the first day that you have missed a period. You may feel slightly tired, nauseous or even pre-menstrual, or you may not notice any changes at all.

week 5 You will probably have noticed that your period is late now. If you did have a period, it will probably have been much lighter than normal, more like spotting. Three layers of cells are developing in the tiny embryo now. The inner layer will form some of the internal organs, the middle layer will form muscles, bones and blood vessels, and the outer layer will form the skin, hair, eyes, nervous system and ears.

week 6 You will have begun to notice changes in your body. Your metabolism is speeding up to deal with the changes that are going on, and you may well feel a little tired as a result. Your uterus is growing and is the size of a tennis ball. Your baby now has a distinct head, the skeleton is forming and buds, which will become arms and legs, have appeared. There is a tiny heart beating and the liver and kidneys, as well as nerve cells, are beginning to develop.

week 7 The baby's cerebral hemispheres are forming and growing. The early-stage limbs are developing clefted fins, which will go on to become fingers and toes. The digestive tract and pancreas are beginning to form.

week 8 The baby is big enough now to mean that your uterus needs to start expanding and you may experience this as a slight cramping feeling. The baby's face is recognisable with a nose tip, a mouth with a little tongue and folds for the eyelids. All the main organs are now in place, the eyes are becoming recognisable, and the arm and legs are developing forwards. An ultrasound may be able to detect if you are pregnant with twins (or more!).

week 9 While you still cannot feel your baby moving, an ultrasound scan may pick up some gentle movements. The baby's head is becoming more distinct with a neck, and the arms and legs are getting longer with hands flexed at the wrists.

week 10 Your baby is now moving its arms and legs in the amniotic fluid. The early stage of the placenta, the chorionic villi, is growing and maturing.

week 11   Male and female sexual characteristics are now beginning to appear. You may be feeling some relief from any morning sickness you have been experiencing.

week 12   Your uterus will now be large enough to push out above your pubic bone. All your baby's fingers and toes (which you will eventually be kissing and nibbling) have now separated and are getting longer. The face is properly formed, and your baby can open and close its mouth. The baby is now fully formed and has now passed the stage when it is most susceptible to damage.

week 13   You are probably noticing a small bump developing. Your baby has no layer of fat and the skin looks quite transparent. The intestines are already beginning to function in a fairly mature way. By the end of the first trimester the placenta has formed fully.

size of your baby in the first trimester

3 weeks	a cluster of cells smaller than a pin tip
5 weeks	2 mm long (the size of an apple pip)
6 weeks	about the size of a watermelon pip
7 weeks	pea sized
8 weeks	2.5 cm – like an olive
9 weeks	the size of a small strawberry
10 weeks	plum-sized
11 weeks	already the size of a medium tomato
12 weeks	6.5 cm long, 12 g in weight and kiwi-sized
13 weeks	a peach!

THE PLACENTA

The placenta is the connecting link between you and your baby. As well as delivering nutrients and oxygen to your baby, it carries away waste products and carbon dioxide. The placenta is also a hormone producing organ and takes over the job of manufacturing sufficient progesterone and oestrogen to keep the pregnancy going. It stores glycogen, which is a ready source of energy, and also makes every known human enzyme.

The early stage of the placenta consists of the chorionic villi, which then grow into the pancake shaped organ that is the placenta. A well developed placenta eventually grows to a weight of between 675–900 g/1½–2 lb. It connects to your baby through the umbilical cord, and endless fun can be had, in later years, telling your incredulous child about how you were both linked up from a rope that went to his or her belly-button!

One of the unique features of the placenta is that it is endowed with two separate blood supplies, the mother's and the baby's. These two blood networks communicate with, but never touch each other. The blood pools between them and there is an exchange of nutrients, gases and waste products. The placenta also acts as a semi-permeable membrane which keeps some harmful substances away from the baby, for example some bacteria. It is not a true barrier, however, and cannot protect the baby from the majority of toxins, so substances such as lead and cadmium, as well as many others, can get through. This is why it is so important to reduce your exposure to anything that might affect your baby. It is not the degree of toxicity that determines whether a substance can get across to the baby, but the size and chemical structure of molecules. Substances such as alcohol, many drugs, and even vitamins A and D in excess, can accumulate to toxic levels in the baby if the mother's levels remain raised. Smoking affects placental health by encouraging calcification of the placental tissue.

The diameter of the blood vessels where the placenta attaches to the uterus become four times bigger. This is equivalent to a garden hose becoming as wide as a large can. During pre-eclampsia the blood vessels do not expand as much and there is reduced blood flow to the baby. Pressure builds up in the mother's blood system, and one school of thought is that the mother is compensating for the narrow vessels by increasing her blood pressure in an attempt to push blood and nutrients through to the baby.

The size, and therefore the performance of the placenta, is directly related to the nourishment of the mother. Even marginal nutrient deficiencies can have a significant effect on its functioning, which in turn affects the baby's development.

POSSIBLE CONCERNS IN THE FIRST TRIMESTER AND THEIR SOLUTIONS

Not all problems have a nutritional basis, or can be corrected with nutrition, but an awful lot can. If you are at all concerned about any symptoms, particularly if they persist, you must consult your doctor. Certainly knowing what to do to support yourself through the three trimesters can make a considerable difference to how you feel during your pregnancy. I have grouped the possible concerns, and what to do about them, under trimesters for ease of reference, but remember that the timing of possible events such as these can be fluid and vary from woman to woman.

Bleeding Gums

This is a problem that can become worse during pregnancy as gums become softer due to the influence of raised progesterone levels, which softens connective tissue. It does this to soften ligaments and muscles in readiness for delivery, but dental health may also be affected. Because the gums are softer, this can increase the chance of gum inflammation, gum disease and tooth decay. The risk of dental caries also increases, as the baby uses up calcium if the mother is not absorbing enough calcium from her diet. Good oral hygiene therefore becomes doubly important. Visit your dentist at least once during pregnancy to have your teeth professionally cleaned and to have a check up. Remember to tell your dentist that you are pregnant, as you need to avoid X-rays and anaesthetics. You also need to avoid amalgam fillings during pregnancy as the effects of mercury on the unborn child can be severe in some cases. You are entitled to free National Health dental checks and treatment while you are pregnant and for the first year after pregnancy.

A mineral rich diet is important in helping to maintain the health of your teeth during pregnancy. Concentrating on foods which are rich in calcium, magnesium and vitamin D can help to maintain tooth and bone health throughout the pregnancy (see **Vitamins and Minerals Needed for a Healthy Pregnancy**, page 73). Nutrients that can help to maintain gum health, and which are safe in pregnancy at the recommended levels, are vitamin C and Co-enzyme Q10. Vitamin C is used to build healthy collagen and bleeding gums is a typical sign, when not pregnant, of mild scurvy, which is caused by vitamin C deficiency. Taking 500–1,000 mg of vitamin C daily can help to maintain oral health. Co-enzyme Q10 (also called Co-Q10 and ubiquinone) is used by all cells for energy manufacture, and it seems to help avoid 'pink-toothbush' at levels of around 60–100 mg daily.

Breast Care

A missed period may not be the first noticeable sign that you are pregnant – it could be changes in your breasts which alert you.

Even in the first few weeks of pregnancy your breasts are already preparing for their role of feeding your infant. You may have mixed feelings about the changing form of your breasts. On the positive side they will not be subject to the monthly hormonal influences which can be uncomfortable for many women, and your bountiful female form may be a source of great pleasure. On the negative side, you may find that you have two aliens developing on your chest. The pink or brown circles around your nipples, called the areolae, will enlarge, become darker in colour and the little bumps called Montgomery's tubercles will become more prominent. Blue lines will also develop around the breasts as the blood supply to the area becomes richer, and your breasts may feel more tender and heavy.

Throughout your pregnancy make sure that your bra fits, and that it does not 'dig-in' to surrounding tissue. Go to a shop with a proper bra-fitter, such as the lingerie department of a department store, and make sure that the bras you use keep pace with your breast development throughout your pregnancy.

One of the things that usually flies out of the window during pregnancy is a regular monthly breast check. As the breasts are changing so much you may think it is impossible to carry out a breast check accurately, particularly since the monthly reminder of your periods is missing. It may seem a bit of a downer starting with this subject, but the reality is that a significant minority of breast cancers are found during pregnancy. Breast cancer is a bit of a bandwagon of mine and I know of no other pregnancy books that mention the subject, so I feel justified in including one paragraph here – if it saves one life it is worth it. The only reason that the prognosis is sometimes worse for women who find they have breast cancer during their pregnancy than it is for others, is that the irregularities are found at a later stage because regular checks have not been done. It is wise to carry on with your breast checks during pregnancy and to report to your doctor any changes to your breast tissue, or the surrounding area, which you do not feel are normal for you or your pregnancy. Check your breasts, the area under the arm and over your collar bone – you could be looking for a lump, an eczema-like rash on the skin or nipple (especially one-sided), an inverted nipple which was not inverted previously, one-sided nipple discharge, puckering of the skin or unusual bruising, swelling or soreness.

Catching a Cold or the Flu

If you are unlucky enough to come down with a bug during your pregnancy do not worry that it will affect your baby. However, in order to be sure that you are not developing symptoms of another disease, it is wise to check with your doctor. As long as you have steered clear of other people with possible infections you should be fine (see **Avoiding Infections**, page 30). If you have children at school, ask the school to tell you immediately if they know of your child coming in to contact with another family which has a disease that you need to avoid.

When you do come down with something it is important not to reach automatically for whatever you have in the medicine cabinet as many drugs can affect the developing baby, including aspirin and mega-doses of vitamins. In any event, taking medication will not cure a cold (a fortune awaits the person who discovers what will), and at best will only relieve and shorten symptoms. The answer is to look after yourself well so that it does not develop into anything worse, such as bronchitis.

Make sure you get extra rest and, if possible, go to bed. Keep eating healthily, and don't be tempted to starve a cold – pregnancy is no time to fast. If you find you don't have much appetite, try eating comforting, easy food such as nourishing soups, fruit smoothies made in a blender or yoghurt desserts.

Drink loads and loads of water and other nourishing fluids to
stay hydrated. If you are running a temperature, or even if you
are just sniffling and sneezing, you will be losing fluids. Make
sure you eat a couple of pieces of citrus fruit or some red berries
such as blackcurrants, or squeeze lemon or orange juice into
water to drink, to maintain your levels of vitamin C. A comforting, immunity supporting broth can be made with a crushed
garlic clove, miso and lemon. A sore throat responds well to that
old standby – lemon and honey with hot water (but without the
shot of whisky!). If you are feverish you can help bring down
your temperature by using cold compresses, having cool sponge
baths, or taking a lukewarm or cool shower. Call your doctor
immediately if you have a temperature approaching 102 degrees
F/40 degrees C. If you have signs of infection, such as coughing
up greenish or yellowish phlegm, call your doctor.

One of the best ways of ensuring that you remain resistant
to colds and infections is to support yourself nutritionally.
One of the points of pre-conceptual planning, apart from ensuring a healthy baby, is to reduce the number of times that a pregnant woman succumbs to health problems. If you manage
to stay infection free during your pregnancy it will be a much
happier one.

Depression and Mood Swings

Pregnancy is a time of fluctuating hormones, and while it might
be irritating to be told 'it's your hormones dear', there is a grain
of truth in this. If you do not normally experience emotional
swings, and find that they become a feature of your pregnancy,
hormones may well be at the root. Apart from anything else,
women are generally expected to be happy about their expectant condition and this may simply not be the way you feel.
You may have all sorts of mixed emotions about your changing

body, about the impact that your pregnancy will have on your relationship with your partner, about how you might be as a mother, as well as anxieties about the health of your baby and any financial pressures caused by the expected arrival.

Eating for a Perfect Pregnancy is designed to even out blood sugar levels which can contribute to mood swing problems. Sugar, coffee, chocolate and alcohol can all play havoc with blood sugar regulation and avoiding these will help to stabilise the brain chemical, serotonin, and beta-endorphins. It is possible for some mild emotional problems to be worsened by deficiencies in one nutrient or another and, if there is depression in the family, you may find that pregnancy exacerbates any nutrient deficiency and pushes you into depression when you might otherwise be OK. Pregnancy is not the time to start experimenting with supplements to correct these deficiencies, instead eating a balanced diet, concentrating on zinc and magnesium rich foods and taking a daily pregnancy formula that includes the B-complex, is the wisest course of action.

Sometimes exercise, particularly slow meditative exercise such as yoga, can help to relieve depression and mood swings. Attending meditation classes can be highly beneficial and can help raise alpha waves (which are associated with calmness) in the brain. Stretching exercises and walking in a lovely place, such as a park, can also be of enormous help.

On no account be tempted to take anti-depressants, unless prescribed by your doctor, and do not take herbal anti-depressant remedies either. If your mood swings or depression seem to be getting more serious it is important to talk either to a counsellor, or to a friend with whom you feel comfortable. In an ideal world your partner would be the person to speak to, but you may have a mate who is either not supportive or to whom you do not feel able to confide. It is important to seek out this sort of help if you need it because, if you continue to feel low, you may not take the best care of yourself or of your baby, which may just make you feel even worse about yourself and perpetuate the vicious spiral.

Digestive Problems

constipation This is a common complaint during pregnancy as the hormone progesterone relaxes the gut muscles. In later pregnancy the growing baby increasingly presses on the mother's internal organs, including her digestive tract and colon. Pregnancy can therefore exacerbate any existing problem. The most important advice is to keep fibre levels high with a varied diet, as described in **Eating for a Perfect Pregnancy**, page 68, and to drink sufficient water on a daily basis. It also helps to avoid dehydrating drinks such as alcohol, coffee and strong tea. An excess of milk and dairy foods is also often linked to constipation. Fibre rich foods that are of particular help include porridge oats, pears, figs, dried apricots and prunes. Eating a variety of fruit, vegetables, pulses, beans and wholegrains is the best policy for avoiding constipation. If baking is something you enjoy add ground linseeds for fibre, or make bran muffins sweetened with dates. If pulses make you 'windy' introduce them slowly into your diet, but do start eating these fibre and mineral rich foods (some ideas include lentil soup, chickpea curry, flageolet beans in vinaigrette, 'home' baked beans, Mexican refried beans). Finally, the physiologically normal way to go to the lavatory is to squat since this position aids comfortable bowel movements. To simulate this position use an upturned wastepaper basket to rest your feet on while you are on the lavatory.

One of the most useful remedies for constipation is to take one or two heaped teaspoons of psyllium husks daily. Take half the amount in the morning and half in the evening, stirred into a cup of fruit juice. Psyllium husks taste like sawdust, but the fruit juice helps them go down (let them swell a little in the juice). Drink another large glass of water after taking the psyllium. This should ensure that your stools are bulky, soft and easy to pass. If you have been constipated for a while or are unused to a lot of fibre in your diet, it may be best to introduce the psyllium into your regime over a couple of weeks, starting with a half teaspoonful and building up.

diarrhoea If you experience diarrhoea, you must keep your water intake up to replace lost fluids. The problem may be caused by an infection or a virus and if you get persistent diarrhoea at any time during your pregnancy you must consult your doctor, as an infection could put your baby at risk.

If you generally err on the side of loose stools, this may be a sign that you need more fibre and the advice above about psyllium husks is just as relevent for loose stools as for constipation. This is because psyllium, and in fact any fibre, acts to regulate bowel movements, not to specifically speed them up or slow them down. Another possible cause of persistently loose stools can be a sensitivity to a food, most usually wheat or dairy products. Going on an exclusion diet (where you eliminate a whole food group) is not recommended during pregnancy as you need to eat sensibly to nourish your baby. Nevertheless, there is no harm in replacing one member of a food group with another of equal nutritional value. For more information about this see pages 57 and 64.

bloating and flatulence The most common reasons for trapped wind or flatulence are constipation and reactions to foods, quite often wheat or dairy products. For constipation see the information above, and for information about other foods that you can eat instead of wheat or dairy products see the relevant sections in **The Food Pyramid**, pages 57 and 64. Flatulence may also be linked to an imbalance of bacteria in your bowels and this can be helped by eating live yoghurt or supplementing with acidophilus supplements (beneficial bacteria), as well as improving fibre levels as described above. Make sure that any acidophilus supplement you buy is stored in the refrigerator and that it guarantees at least 1 billion viable organisms.

indigestion   Indigestion or heartburn are more common in the later stages of the pregnancy (see **Heartburn**, page 174). However, if you suffer from indigestion earlier on you will need to avoid antacids and many herbal remedies, including aloe vera. Herbal teas that can be helpful in settling indigestion, and which are safe in pregnancy, are mint, camomile and ginger (see **The Natural Remedy Cupboard**, page 119). Sometimes dealing with indigestion can be as simple as eating smaller meals – have five small meals during the day instead of three large ones. Treat yourself to regular starters or puddings of fresh papaya or pineapple as these two fruits are extremely high in digestive enzymes that can help to reduce problems with indigestion.

Fatigue

Feeling like lying down from time to time is perfectly natural and is Mother Nature's way of telling you to ease up a little. Everyone's experience of pregnancy is different, and it is not a competition. Because your neighbour or sister sailed through a pregnancy with all the energy in the world is no reason to think that you 'ought' to as well.

Fatigue is more common in the first trimester, and the good news is that the second trimester usually brings relief. The reason why the first third of the pregnancy may be worse for fatigue may be that there are profound metabolic changes going on which take a while for your body to get used to. Not only are you starting and growing a life, but your whole body is undergoing changes such as building up breast tissue, building up the uterus, increasing your blood volume, raising levels of hormones, and building up a placenta.

The hormone progesterone, levels of which increase in the first three months, has a sedative effect. This can be beneficial in making a woman more relaxed in the face of forthcoming events (she needs to be, she has to squeeze a large watermelon sized baby out of a small tube — of course she has to stay calm!).

It is also common for sleeping patterns to be disturbed, and to experience some nausea and mood swings, all of which can make the problem of fatigue worse.

If you are feeling really knocked out, you may need to pay greater attention to your eating habits. If you are still eating sugary foods, which give a quick burst of energy and then lead to a dip in blood sugar levels sufficient to make you feel like falling asleep, this is a hint that you need to substitute foods that serve you better. Concentrate on eating a little protein along with some complex carbohydrates at each meal. Eat regularly, say every four hours, and make sure your snacks are nutritious ones such as fruit, yoghurt, half a stuffed wholemeal pitta bread, oatcakes or rye crackers with a spread or a handful of fresh nuts. This will help keep your blood sugar levels even and give you fuel that will burn for several hours, not several minutes.

If you are unnaturally fatigued, this can be a sign that your blood iron levels are low and you need to ask your doctor for a blood test to detect anaemia.

Relaxation classes, yoga and meditation can all be beneficial in reducing fatigue and improving sleeping patterns. If there is a time of day when you regularly experience fatigue, plan around it. Don't push yourself too hard, enjoy the fact that you have an excuse to coddle yourself, and take a nap if you need and want to.

Food Cravings and Aversions

It is not uncommon for women to find that they develop food cravings during pregnancy or aversions to favourite foods, particularly in the first three months. Sometimes the combinations craved can be very strange indeed – jam and pickle sandwiches or sardines with bananas. Sometimes the cravings are attributed to particular nutrient deficiencies that the woman may have. Iron deficiency may trigger a taste for red meat, calcium deficiency may make you strangely attracted to chalk, zinc deficiency may make you crave oysters. It is more likely, however, that the cravings are linked to changes in hormone levels, which affect saliva and make some foods taste different from the way they usually do. It is often the case that strong tasting foods are craved because pregnancy dulls the taste buds.

Despite stories of strange food cravings and combinations of foods, the most commonly craved foods are fruit, vegetables, confectionery, cereal products and fish. This rather suggests that cravings are centred around the healthier options (other than confectionery, which is a likely sign of blood sugar imbalance). Unless the craved food causes indigestion, or is extremely low in nutrients, there is no harm in indulging yourself. Common sense can be applied to all of this, and if you find that you can't face vegetables or other healthy foods you normally eat, maybe this is the time to get creative with your cooking. On the other hand, if the smell of coffee is making you gag, that is just fine – don't fight it. If you find that nausea or aversion to food is leading to you eating insufficient amounts of food, maybe because you can't face a full meal, you may have to think of ways to overcome this. Don't worry if your aversion is to milk or milky foods. Milk is hugely overrated in pregnancy and is often suggested as a source of calcium because people do not know what else contains this mineral. If you find that you can't tolerate dairy products, see **The Calcium Question**, page 73.

If you find that you are reaching for energy 'props' such as ice cream and biscuits, read the sections on **Junk Food Junkies**, page 112, and **Gestational Diabetes**, page 116. In pre-packet-of-biscuit days, if people craved carbohydrates for energy they had no option but to reach for fruit, berries, grains, nuts or pulses. The availability of convenience snack foods sabotages healthy eating plans and makes decision making all the more difficult if you are driven by strong cravings. Luckily, by the second trimester food cravings and aversions tend to disappear for most women.

Sometimes women are affected by a condition called pica. This is when you find you are strangely attracted to eating clay, ashes, chalk, charcoal or detergents. This should be reported to your doctor as it can be a sign of mineral deficiencies, particularly iron.

Frequent Urination and Cystitis

It is common in pregnancy to find yourself running off for a pee more often than usual, most typically in the first trimester and in the last. This is caused by an increase in body fluids and because the kidneys are working more efficiently to eliminate waste products. The pressure of the uterus on the bladder is another factor, though this is partially relieved in the second trimester as the uterus rises up into the higher part of the abdominal cavity. Of course, everyone's internal organs are arranged slightly differently, so if you do not find that you have an increase in the pattern of your urination don't let that be a source of concern!

In later months the problem often returns as the baby drops into a lower position again. This can be particularly irritating at night when you are hoping for unbroken sleep. The only real remedy is to avoid drinking liquids after, say, 6 pm at night. However, still make sure that you maintain your overall fluid intake (at least 2 litres/8 large glasses daily).

If the need to urinate is accompanied by a burning sensation, you may have cystitis. If so, cut out sugar and sugary foods from your diet, drink plenty of water, drink 1 litre/1¾ pints of cranberry juice or unsweetened lemon juice diluted with water daily and make sure you take your 1 gram of vitamin C daily. Some people find that cranberry pills are even more effective than the juice, as the latter usually comes with a hefty load of sugar. Drink cornsilk tea to reduce pain and soothe the urinary tract, or use dandelion leaf tea. Burdock tincture (25–30 drops in water three times daily) helps to heal an irritated urinary tract. An alkaline based drink such as sodium bicarbonate and sodium citrate can also help, as can eating live yoghurt as it is a source of beneficial bacteria that help protect against cystitis and thrush. Spend time on the lavatory making sure that you empty your bladder fully (leaning forward helps); make sure, too, that your underwear is of cotton rather than synthetic material, and that your clothes are loose fitting. Don't put off going to the lavatory either, as people who 'hold it in' are more susceptible to infections. Finally, avoid perfumed soaps, powders and bath essences on the area.

If cystitis persists or is very uncomfortable refer to your doctor immediately as infections can travel up the urinary tract and lead to more serious infections in the bladder and kidneys and can affect the pregnancy.

Headaches

It is frequently the case that headaches become worse during pregnancy. Headaches are linked to many factors, including stress and neck and back tensions. Nutritionally speaking you need to make sure that you are not constipated, dehydrated or experiencing dips in blood sugar levels, all of which are major contributing factors to headaches. Your headaches may also be triggered by certain foods, the most common culprits being chocolate, oranges, coffee, red wine, dairy products (especially if you also suffer from blocked sinuses) and wheat products. Headaches may also be a sign of iron, calcium or magnesium deficiency. Herbs that can be helpful in clearing headaches are camomile, lemon balm, meadowsweet and lavender. If you experience a sudden onset of headaches after the fifth or sixth month then consult your doctor as this may be a sign of pre-eclampsia.

Morning (Noon and Night) Sickness

Morning sickness is a misnomer because feeling nauseous can come at any time of the day or night, so let's call it pregnancy sickness. It can be made worse by any number of things, most usually the smell of certain foods. If it happens more frequently in the morning, it may be because of low blood sugar levels. One-third to one-half of women experience pregnancy sickness. While pregnancy sickness seems to be worse in the first three months, it is also possible for the nausea to continue into later months, or to disappear and then return later. Sometimes the first time a woman suspects she may be pregnant is because she is feeling nauseous.

Some women experience ptyalism, an excess of saliva, often associated with morning sickness, but this usually disappears in the second trimester. You may find that it helps to brush your teeth more frequently, suck on a mint or chew gum.

Interestingly, a study in Sweden seems to confirm the old wives' tale that women who experience more intense sickness are more likely to give birth to girls. This is thought to be because the hormones that a baby girl produces affect the mother's hormone balance – the extra oestrogens serve to top up the mother's. Conversely, the male hormones that a little boy produces serve to act as a counterbalance to the mother's and may lead to less instances of morning sickness. However, this is far from a reliable method of predicting the sex of your unborn baby, because the quantity of the various hormones the baby produces can be variable, and the effect probably depends upon the mother's own initial hormone status.

Pregnancy sickness rarely leads to a diet being so restricted, or food being vomited so much, that it becomes a danger to the pregnancy, yet you obviously have to make sure you are eating a nutritious diet and not avoiding too many foods. It may be helpful to eat little snacky meals instead of larger ones. Stress may have a large part to play in morning sickness since women who are relieved of the burdens of daily life (work, families, inability to rest, worries) are more able to overcome the problem, as has been demonstrated in women who are hospitalised with what is called hyperemesis or excessive vomiting. Nausea is more common in first pregnancies than in later pregnancies. This may be linked to the physical and emotional assault on the first-time mother, who is better prepared on all levels the next time around.

some steps you can take to alleviate morning sickness:

- Eat a diet based on proteins and complex carbohydrates which keeps stimulants and empty calories to a minimum, as described in **Eating for a Perfect Pregnancy**.
- Make sure you maintain your fluid intake, especially if you are losing liquid when you vomit.
- Make sure that you take your pregnancy-formulated

supplement at a time when you are not likely to throw it up. There is some evidence that taking moderate supplement doses that include vitamin B6 helps reduce pregnancy sickness symptoms.

- Avoid smells that nauseate you, and don't even look at foods which may trigger an attack. Don't make yourself eat foods that make you feel queasy, and don't feel the need to make these foods for your family.

- Eat little and often, if necessary before you really feel hungry. Low blood sugar levels can trigger nausea faster than anything else. If necessary keep a snack by your bed to avoid blood sugar lows in the middle of the night or in the morning – a banana or a couple of oatcakes are ideal.

- Don't conform to normal meal-time expectations if you don't want to. If you crave sweeter foods, then wholemeal pancakes with fruit for supper is just fine. Conversely, if savouries are your thing, a tuna-melt sandwich on wholewheat for breakfast works just as well as the more normal muesli with dried fruit and juice.

- Don't feel bad about your morning sickness, as this will only serve to increase your anxiety levels, and remember your baby is unlikely to be affected by it. Explain to your partner and workmates what is going on.

- Take a break when you need it. As already mentioned, stress is closely linked to morning sickness. If you can, take it easy when you get up in the morning, and have a cup of soothing peppermint tea.

- Eat easy-to-digest foods such as yoghurt, fruit and juices, steamed fish, soups and steamed vegetables.

- Avoid bending forward as this can stimulate the vagus nerve leading to the stomach.

- Clean out your refrigerator of all foods that make you feel queasy.

- Avoid travelling wherever possible, as motion and fumes can make you feel worse.
- Brushing your teeth or sucking on a mint helps some women, as does drinking sparkling mineral water.
- Chemists stock acupressure wrist-bands that are designed to help relieve morning sickness and motion sickness. They work on acupuncture point PC6 (about two thumb widths above the crease of your wrist on the front of your fore-arm – which you could also press with your thumb). This is not recommended after the eighth week of pregnancy. Morning sickness also responds well to acupuncture.
- Consult a homeopath, as remedies such as nux vomica, pulsatilla and sepica can be effective.

ginger and fennel drink

Ginger is one of the oldest remedies for nausea and has been shown in trials to be highly effective. Keep a peeled ginger root in your freezer so that it is always on hand. Slice off shavings or cubes as you need it. Fennel is used for colic, lowering intestinal wind and calming a queasy stomach.

recipe for one large glass: ½ head of fennel, 100 ml/4 fl oz filtered water, 1 tsp ginger root. Wash the fennel and place in a juicer with the ginger, then add the water.

If you do not have ginger tea or ginger and fennel drink to hand, other options are good quality ginger biscuits, ginger ale, crystallised ginger, ginger syrup or ginger capsules.

Thrush

If you have a light white discharge without accompanying itch-ing it is unlikely to be thrush. A light discharge is normal during pregnancy (similar to that which most women get in the days before their period) and it increases in amount throughout pregnancy. It can be copious enough for some women to feel they need to wear a pad towards the end of their pregnancy. If, on the other hand, you develop a thick whitish or yellowish vaginal discharge, which may have a foul odour, and may be accompanied by vaginal itching, you could have thrush (monilia or candida albicans), bacterial vaginosis or some other infection.

Hormonal changes during pregnancy make women 10 to 20 times more susceptible to thrush infections. Thrush can strike at any time during the pregnancy. Early on it is no more than an irritation, but your doctor will want to make sure that any infection is cleared up if it happens near to delivery time to avoid the baby getting thrush.

There are several things you can do to reduce the likelihood of getting an attack of thrush. Avoid sugar, sugary foods, refined carbohydrates and alcohol and increase garlic, live yoghurt, ginger and olive oil in your diet, as these have a beneficial effect. Drink plenty of water, and also take an acidophilus (beneficial bacteria) supplement daily (buy a supplement with at least one billion viable organisms and keep it in the refrigerator). You should not use any dietary, herbal or other anti-candida supplements while you are pregnant. Nor should you use douches, and in particular douche-syringes, as they can lead to a life-threatening air embolism.

You can, however, bathe the outer genital area with live yoghurt. Let the yoghurt come to room temperature, scoop out as much yeast as you are able from your vagina using your two middle fingers, wash your hands and then smear the yoghurt into all the creases and up into the vaginal tract only as far as your fingers will go. Repeat twice daily during an acute infection, and twice a week if you are prone to infections. You can also use an acidophilus capsule as a night suppository. (This works if the environment is alkaline, but can aggravate it if it is already acidic. If this is the case, use two tablespoons of baking soda in a cup of warm water.) A pessary of a garlic clove is also highly effective, but when you peel the garlic clove make sure that you do not scratch the clove surface or it will sting unmercifully. Other solutions to use on the outer genital area only are a few drops of tea tree oil diluted in water, a quarter cup of apple cider vinegar diluted in ¾ cup of warm water, a lavender infusion or aloe vera gel.

Wear cotton rather than man-made fibres for your underwear. Consult your doctor if the infection persists, but do not buy over-the-counter oral anti-thrush medication if you are pregnant or if you are breast-feeding.

Water Retention (Oedema)

This is most often a problem during the second half of pregnancy, although as some women experience bloating earlier on I have included it in this section. Hormonal changes during pregnancy can increase the likelihood of sodium retention and it is therefore wise to keep your salt intake to a sensible level. We need around 6 g of salt daily, but most people eat between 9 g and 12 g. While it is helpful not to add salt to your food at the table, or when you are cooking, we get by far the most salt from packaged foods. It is not even obviously salty foods, such as crisps, that necessarily tot up our salt levels, but everyday food items such as bread and cereals. Do not be tempted to go on a salt-free diet as we need some salt – it is excess that leads to problems.

Here is an abbreviated list of the salt content of common foods to help you to keep to 6 g daily. For other packaged foods check the labels for the amount of sodium per 100 g or per portion. To convert the sodium listed on the package into grams of salt, multiply the sodium figure by 2.5. Therefore 0.4 g of sodium is equal to 1 g of salt.

bacon, 2 rashers back bacon (55 g)	2.5 g
baked beans (200 g)	2.5 g
baking powder (1 level teaspoon)	1.3 g
Bovril (1 tsp)	0.5 g
bread, medium slice	0.5 g
burger or beanburger, and fries	3.0–6.0 g
butter, salted (20 g – average for two slices)	0.4 g
cereal, bowl (40 g serving)	0.9–1.5 g
cheese, hard (55 g)	1.4 g
cheese and tomato pizza, 1 slice (225 g)	5.3 g
cottage cheese (115 g)	1.3 g
crisps, packet (35 g bag)	0.5 g
salt (1 level teaspoon)	5.0 g
sausages, pork 2 (115 g)	3.4 g
sea salt (1 level teaspoon)	3.5 g
soup, canned – 1 bowl (250 ml)	2.5 g
soy sauce (1 level tablespoon)	3.6 g
stock cube (½ cube)	0.9 g
tomato juice (250 ml)	1.4 g
tomato ketchup, 1 sachet (25 g)	0.8 g

Just as important as being sensible about sodium levels is making sure you get enough potassium in your diet by eating lots of fruit and vegetables. Potassium helps to balance out sodium levels. To keep water retention under control it is also helpful to ensure that you are drinking your 2 litres/3½ pints of water a day – clean water is vital to flush out 'stagnant' water. If you have less than perfect bowel movements see Constipation, page 140, to help to keep waste products moving out of your body and so avoid them encouraging water retention. One pregnant lady I know had the most terrible water retention early in her pregnancy, which was mostly resolved when she stopped drinking 2 litres of diet coke daily and substituted it with hot water with lemon and honey. Oedema can lead to carpal tunnel syndrome as waterlogged tissues press on nerves to the fingers resulting in tingling and numbness. If you get this wear a wrist splint and avoid lying on your arms, or repetitive actions such as typing. Put your feet up regularly to reduce the problem of pooling around the ankles. You may need to put a thick pillow under the foot-end of your mattress. It is essential to keep moving if you experience water retention, as the muscle movements will help to keep lymph flowing around the body for cleansing. Soak your feet in a warm foot bath with ½ cup of Epsom salts and a handful of lavender or rosemary. Use arnica cream or oil. Drink a nettle or dandelion infusion (two cups daily) or take tinctures, 15–20 drops of each twice daily.

If your bloating continues and is getting out of control you must see your doctor, especially if it is in the last half of your pregnancy as it may be a sign of pre-eclampsia (see page 161).

CHAPTER SIX

The Second Trimester

· ·

For most people this is when the fun really starts. If you have been feeling queasy or tired, this is usually when you begin to feel a whole lot better. You, and maybe your partner, might have taken a little while to get used to the idea that you are pregnant and all the changes that this will make to your life, but now you might be settling down to enjoy the experience. You will begin to have a bump showing which, if you have put off telling people before, means that you are likely to start letting everyone know that you are expecting a bundle of joy. The goodwill that this usually engenders is something to capitalise on. People are often amazingly helpful from now until a few weeks after the birth, but later, when you really need their help because your little bundle of cuddles won't sleep through the night, you'll often find that everyone around you seems to think that it is business as usual. So take advantage of all the goodwill now!

WHAT IS HAPPENING TO YOU AND YOUR BABY

week 14 You will hopefully be turning a corner in terms of how you feel. You should not now feel quite so tired and any morning sickness you have been experiencing should recede. The reason that you begin to feel more lively is that the baby is now mature enough to produce adrenaline and you are reaping the benefits of this. Some hair has now grown on your baby's head and eyebrows have formed. The baby will move in response to stimuli, such as noise and light, and responds to touch.

week 15 The soft cartilaginous tissue that makes up your baby's bones will be starting to harden. You might experience some period-like pains in your lower abdomen which give you cause for concern, but this is normal and does not mean that anything is amiss. Provided it is not accompanied by any bleeding, then it is just the strange sensation of your uterus expanding.

week 16 Your baby's limbs are now fully formed and being put to good use – you may possibly begin to sense a slight fluttering in your abdomen (this is more likely if this is your second or later baby, if it is your first it is more common to feel movement at 18–20 weeks). A soft, downy hair, called lanugo, is forming all over the baby, including over the face.

week 17 Your baby has individual fingerprints, its finger- and toenails are growing and it already has a firm handgrip.

week 18 The lungs are now being developed by the process of the baby breathing in, or gulping, amniotic fluid. If you have an ultrasound around this time you may spot your baby already sucking its thumb.

week 19 Buds for your baby's permanent adult teeth are forming behind those that have already formed for milk teeth. Your waistline is beginning to expand and your navel may well be flattening out.

week 20 You are halfway through the pregnancy now, and you should be able to feel distinct movements. The baby's muscles are developing rapidly allowing for more energetic movements.

week 21 The top of your uterus has moved high enough to be parallel with your belly button. The baby is still small enough to move around freely in the amniotic fluid and its kicking will be getting stronger. You may even discern a pattern of movement at certain times of the day or night and during quiet times your baby may be asleep.

week 22 Your baby's digestive tract is working in a basic manner. Undigested amniotic fluid will pass into your baby's bowels, and eventually be excreted as meconium after the birth.

week 23 You will probably have put on between 4.5–6.8 kg/10–15 lb. With a little practice you may be able to work out the different parts of your baby through your abdominal wall. Your baby weighs around 450 g/1 lb and looks like a little doll. The brain cells are becoming increasingly inter-linked and 'branched'. Your baby is able to respond to familiar voices and music and will turn away from very bright lights.

week 24 Your baby's brain is becoming sufficiently wired up for the baby to be aware of pain. Your baby looks more like a full-term baby already, but while its vital organs are functioning the lungs are not sufficiently developed to manage on its own.

week 25 The baby has developed a 'righting' reflex already and knows which way is up and which is down. You will be aware of when your baby is asleep or awake if you pay attention to its movements. This will not always coincide with your own patterns and he or she may be doing football practice when you are trying to sleep.

week 26 Your baby is putting on weight at a tremendous rate and now weighs around 900 g/2lb. The typical transparency of developing babies is being lost as fat layers build up under the skin. Your baby can open its eyes for the first time and, if born, would have a good chance of survival in a premature baby unit.

size of your baby in the second trimester

15 weeks	a large avocado
16 weeks	a grapefruit
18 weeks	a cantaloupe melon
20 weeks	a honeydew melon
24 weeks	a small watermelon

POSSIBLE CONCERNS IN THE SECOND TRIMESTER AND THEIR SOLUTIONS

Allergies

It is common in pregnancy to find that nasal 'stuffiness' is made worse. On the other hand, women who regularly suffer from allergies may find that pregnancy eases the symptoms as their immune system is 'tuned down' to avoid reacting to the baby, and levels of the hormones cortisone and adrenaline increase slightly. If you find that you are uncharacteristically stuffed-up it may not be an allergy at all, but the result of increased blood flow to the nasal membranes, under the influence of rising pregnancy hormone levels, making them softer and more swollen. It is also more common to have nose bleeds during pregnancy, for the same reasons. You may also be eating more foods, such as dairy products, in the interest of eating healthily, and are finding that they are actually causing a bad reaction. If you think this may be the case, see **The Food Pyramid**, page 50, for alternative foods in the same food group that you can substitute for those that may be causing the reaction. Taking 1 g of vitamin C daily can help to strengthen mucous membranes in the nose and may reduce the problem. This multi-purpose

vitamin also acts as a natural antihistamine, so if you are affected by a true allergy it may help. Steam inhalations are a good
way to loosen any mucus.

Anaemia

If you are feeling particularly fatigued and have a pale skin, you
may suspect anaemia. You will be getting regular blood tests at
your antenatal clinic, and if they pick up anaemia they will tell
you. The most common form of anaemia is a deficiency of iron,
which is vital for red blood cell function. Without sufficient
quantities of this mineral the blood is unable to deliver oxygen
to cells and this results in the typical exhaustion, a pale skin or
dizziness.

Anaemia is common in women, pregnant or not, because of
monthly blood loss, coupled with low dietary intake. This means
that many women start their pregnancy low in iron, and one in
five women go on to become anaemic during pregnancy.

When pregnant, a woman's blood volume increases by a
third to a half. This leads to dilution of the red blood cells in the
blood plasma – so while the amount of red blood cells has not
decreased, the dilution in the carrying liquid has changed – this
is called haemodilution. Although a woman's need for iron
increases in pregnancy – an extra 550 mg is needed overall,
300 mg for the baby, 50 mg for the placenta and 200 mg to
compensate for blood loss at delivery – the absorption of iron
from foods is naturally increased, and of course she is no longer
losing iron through monthly bleeding.

If the haemoglobin count is below 11 in mid-pregnancy you
will probably need to boost levels using dietary, supplemental
and herbal means. It is important not to supplement excess iron
unless a blood test has confirmed that you are definitely anaemic,
because excess iron serves to unbalance other minerals that are

vital for a healthy pregnancy and baby, in particular zinc, and may encourage jaundice in the newborn baby.

In the last two months of a pregnancy the baby will store enough iron in its liver, from the mother's supplies, to last it for the first six months of life. This is Mother Nature's clever way of ensuring that the baby has enough, because breast milk is naturally low in iron and most babies begin to eat solids by around six months, which then provides iron from the diet. If the mother is anaemic, however, it is possible for the baby to also start its life anaemic.

A well balanced diet will go a long way towards avoiding the problem of pregnancy related anaemia. The best sources of iron from the diet are red meat, dark turkey meat, eggs, beets, blackstrap molasses, dark green leafy vegetables, pumpkin and sunflower seeds, dried fruit (raisins, prunes, figs, apricots) and alfalfa (in moderation). Seaweeds, and particularly kelp, are also rich sources of iron. In addition to shredding them and adding them to soups and stews, you can buy specially prepared seaweed that can either be sprinkled on foods as flakes or put into a grinder and used as you would salt. In order to maximise your uptake of dietary iron, aim to have a vitamin C rich food or drink with each meal. This could simply be a small glass of orange juice or a portion of fruit or vegetables, such as broccoli. Vitamin C doubles the absorption of iron from non-meat foods. Conversely, the tannins in tea can reduce the uptake of iron from foods by as much as two-thirds, and the phytic acid in the fibre in wheatbran also reduces the uptake of iron. The phosphates found in colas and similar drinks also limit the uptake of iron, and in any event they are detrimental to overall good health. Better to substitute some fresh juice with sparkling or still water, or an iced fruit tea. Cooking in cast iron pots is such an efficient way of improving iron levels that it has been promoted in developing countries where anaemia is rife.

General pregnancy-formulated supplements usually contain 10–20 mg of iron. If you are anaemic your doctor may recommend an iron 'tonic' or iron supplements of between 20–40 mg. If it is suggested that you take more this may not be wise as it can interfere with other nutrients such as zinc and copper. Those with haemachromatosis should not take iron supplements. Many of the supplements suggested can make you constipated, just what you don't need when your guts are so squashed together anyway! If this happens, use a different type of iron – the ferrous, and not ferric, form (for example, ferrous sulphate or iron ascorbate); 20–40 mg will be prescribed by your doctor (100 mg of ferrous sulphate is equivalent to 30 mg of useable iron). Other nutrients are needed to make sure that blood can carry enough oxygen and these are the B-vitamins (particularly B12 and folic acid), vitamin C and essential fats.

Increasing your iron levels using herbs can be very effective. You can take liquid or tablet chlorophyll which is rich in iron. Supplements that are based on beetroot and nettle are useful. Nettle tea acts as an excellent tonic and can be drunk daily throughout pregnancy to prevent anaemia. Steep a large handful of dried leaves in 1 litre/1¾ pints of boiling water for an hour or so. This makes a strong tasting brew. To make a weaker tonic, steep three or four tablespoons in the same amount of water for half an hour. Drink between one and four cups daily, depending on your needs. Floradix can also be a successful way of redressing iron levels when used alongside diet and other herbal recommendations.

Blood Pressure, Pre-eclampsia, Eclampsia

If your blood pressure is abnormally high in pregnancy, this may be a sign of pre-eclampsia. Pre-eclampsia, also called toxaemia, is most common in the final three or four months of a pregnancy and is associated with a poorly functioning placenta. Pre-eclampsia happens most often in first pregnancies, and rarely in second and later pregnancies (unless the pregnancy is by a different partner). The signs that can lead to a suspicion of pre-eclampsia are high blood pressure and fluid retention. Tests will reveal that there is a loss of proteins in the urine. Other symptoms can include headaches, nausea or vomiting, pains in the abdomen and disturbed vision. If the condition is left untreated eclampsia can develop, which is extremely serious and results in seizures. If your partner complains that you are snoring all of a sudden take this seriously, as it may be an early sign of high blood pressure. One in four pregnant women have an increase in snoring by the last trimester and snorers have double the rate of high blood pressure and pre-eclampsia.

Pre-eclampsia happens in around one in ten pregnancies and needs to be treated urgently as it can lead to losing the baby. Mild cases are usually dealt with by prescribing bed-rest, blood pressure lowering drugs and sometimes aspirin. In severe cases the baby may be delivered prematurely by Caesarean section.

There have been some good studies showing that the incidence of pre-eclampsia can be reduced significantly. The most important findings are linked to diet and supplementation:

● Antioxidant supplements taken daily during the second half of pregnancy have cut the incidence of high blood pressure resulting from pre-eclampsia in 76 per cent of the women tested in a significant trial (compared to those taking a placebo). The antioxidants used were vitamin C (1 g) and vitamin E (400 ius) in weeks 16–22. It is thought that this effect is seen because antioxidants quench the damaging activities of free radicals (harmful molecules that attack tissues) on the placenta, allowing it to function more efficiently and promoting healthy blood flow. More free radicals are created on a diet that is high in sugar, refined carbohydrates, hydrogenated fats and alcohol, as well as by smoking. The beauty of the trial above is that it was a classically designed one exploring the effects of a supplement with a given condition, and balanced out by using a placebo. It had remarkably effective results. Of course, such trials need to be repeated, but these levels of vitamins are generally considered safe in pregnancy.

- GLA (gamma-linolenic acid) (450 mg) found in evening primrose oil and borage oil, along with 600 mg of calcium, taken during the last trimester, has been shown in another trial to lower the number of women who developed pre-eclampsia. Several other trials conclude that around 1 g of calcium significantly reduces the incidence of pre-eclampsia.

- Magnesium (300–500 mg daily) can be useful in treating pre-eclampsia, possibly because of its role in normalising the metabolism of calcium (see above).

- One trial, giving women a multivitamin with 10 mg of vitamin B6 found that 1.1 per cent of them developed pre-eclampsia, versus 4.4 per cent of women taking a multivitamin without any added vitamin B6.

- Garlic powder has been shown to have beneficial effects on pre-eclampsia by stimulating improved placental function.

- Low dose aspirin may be recommended by your doctor for pre-eclampsia. Vitamin E, garlic capsules and fish oil capsules may not be advised alongside aspirin as all three compounds have blood thinning effects. Taking 100 ius of vitamin E, a clove of garlic daily and eating oily fish are unlikely to be contra-indicated, unless your doctor is being hyper-cautious, but always check with your physician.

Pre-eclampsia should never be treated solely by nutritional means and if you have any of the signs or symptoms of this condition you must contact your obstetrician. The information above relates to avoiding the condition developing in the first place. However, if you do have pre-eclampsia, and if your doctor is happy to take a wait and see approach, there is no reason not to follow the advice above, as long as your doctor agrees.

Feeling Faint

If you feel faint it is important to listen to what your body is telling you and to take it easy. You can find immediate relief by sitting down and putting your head between your knees. It is often the case that feeling faint is a result of lowered blood pressure, which is a common symptom during pregnancy. When you take a bath, make sure that it is not too hot, and stand up slowly when you get out. Also get up slowly when you have been lying down. If you are aware that low blood pressure tends to be a problem for you (even when not pregnant) you may need to nurture your adrenal glands by learning some stress management techniques. The adrenal glands produce our stress hormones, adrenaline and cortisol, and low levels of these hormones from overtaxed adrenal glands (a result of chronic stress) can contribute to low blood pressure. Poor regulation of blood sugar levels is another likely contributor to bouts of faintness, in which case read up on the information in Junk Food Junkies, page 112, and Gestational Diabetes, page 116.

Forgetfulness

Even the most organised and on-the-ball women need to develop a sense of humour about the forgetfulness that is fairly typical of advancing pregnancy. They might as well see the funny side, because it is likely to continue for the first few months of their baby's life as well. It may have its root in hormonal changes, or just in having too much to do and with interrupted sleep. Additionally research has shown that the brains of many women shrink very slightly in the later stages of pregnancy and do not fully recover until about six months after the baby is born. It is thought that this might happen because the baby uses up fats that make up the mother's brain for its own development, and it takes several months to restore the full quota. If this is correct, then logically it would be beneficial to ensure that you get sufficient essential fats from your diet (see **Essential Fats**, page 53) and in particular, those from oily fish.

Vitamin B rich foods also support brain health because these vitamins are essential for brain function. Deficiency signs include spaciness, forgetfulness and mood swings (sound familiar?). It can help brain function to take a tablespoon of lecithin daily (available from health food shops), which is a rich source of choline, another B-vitamin found in high amounts in the brain.

Muscle Cramps

Muscle cramps are usually related to an altered calcium/magnesium balance, which affects the nerves controlling the muscles. The baby is using up a lot of these minerals and this can increase the incidence of cramps. Eating a diet rich in calcium and magnesium can help, as can, if necessary, supplementing between 300–500 mg of magnesium on its own, or a ratio of 250 mg calcium to 500 mg of magnesium for a couple of months. Garlic and fish oils help blood flow to the muscles, and anti-oxidants, including Co-enzyme Q10, help oxygen use by the muscles. Dehydration can also play a part as it can affect the muscles, so make sure that you maintain your water intake. If you are still smoking, this may be a further sign to stop as one of the effects is to reduce circulation, particularly to the legs. It is also possible that your muscle cramps are related to a salt deficiency, which can occur if you have been on a no-salt diet for a while or are in a hot country where you perspire a lot.

Persistent leg pain, particularly when it is accompanied by a localised heat or swollen veins, may be due to phlebitis (inflammation of the veins). If you suspect this do not massage the area, but instead refer to your doctor.

Stretch Marks

Stretch marks happen when an area of skin is expanded beyond its normal elasticity, either during pregnancy or other weight gain. They start off as red marks, but eventually fade to silvery streaks. It obviously helps to avoid putting on weight too suddenly.

Stretch marks are more common when a person is deficient in zinc. As zinc is such an important mineral for the developing baby, it is likely that the baby is taking as much of the mother's zinc stores as possible, leaving little for skin health. Supplementing with zinc at around 15 mg daily may help to reduce the likelihood of stretch marks developing (see page 76 for more information about zinc during pregnancy). Essential fats are also vital for skin health, and taking a gram or two of evening primrose oil or a tablespoonful of flax oil daily can help to maintain the integrity of the skin. It is important, too, to maintain your vitamin C levels by eating lots of fresh fruit and vegetables, and possibly taking 500–1000 mg of vitamin C, to keep the collagen which glues skin together in peak health. Another helpful measure is to pierce a 400 iu vitamin E capsule and rub the oil on to the skin at the side of your belly, breasts and top of your thighs, where stretch marks might appear, to help prevent them developing. Zinc and vitamin C creams can also be helpful when rubbed into the skin.

Twins or More

Double the pleasure and, of course, double the call on your reserves. The main point to bear in mind from the nutritional standpoint is that multiple births will mean that a mother needs to be even more in tune with her diet to make sure that she is providing all that her babies need. It is important for a mother of multiple babies to look after herself to make sure that she is not nutritionally depleted by the time she has gone to full term. If you have not been taking a prenatal supplement then being told you are carrying twins would be a very good reason to change this policy.

Weight gain is obviously going to be greater with twins, not only because of the babies, but also because of the weight of the placentas, amniotic fluid and so on. About 50 per cent extra weight should generally be allowed for in the case of twins, when compared to single baby pregnancies. There is not enough information about triplet pregnancies (or more!) to give any general guidelines.

Research shows that a high calorie, nutrient dense diet can significantly improve the chances of having healthy twins who are not low weight at birth. You should aim for an extra 500 calories and an extra portion of protein food, though some information suggests an extra 25 g of protein after the 20th week (i.e. 85 g protein instead of 60 g). A good way to get extra protein without hugely increasing the amount of food you eat is to add skimmed milk powder or soya protein powder to a smoothie. The extra calories should not be achieved by eating higher calorie foods just for the sake of it – remember they need to be nutrient dense as well. Instead add more cold-pressed vegetable or olive oil, avocados and nuts, nut butters and seeds to your diet or choose full fat dairy produce in place of the low fat versions. It is a good idea to spread your calorie intake over the whole day, by snacking often, so that you are getting a regular supply of energy.

Varicose Veins and Haemorrhoids

Varicose veins occur when the valves in veins, which ensure the flow of blood in the lower half of the body up towards the heart, collapse at various places. When this happens blood pools in the veins causing bulges. You can see them as blue, knotted veins on your legs, and they can be painful when they swell. Varicose veins are also common in the anal area and are then called haemorrhoids (piles). The pressure of the developing baby during pregnancy can increase the chance of varicose veins and haemorrhoids developing. If you are prone to varicose veins (they can run in families), or put on too much weight during pregnancy, the risk of developing them is greater. Standing for too long can make the problem worse, as can wearing tight clothing with waist bands that dig in. Whenever possible rest with your feet up for half an hour and wear support tights.

To help reduce the risk of developing haemorrhoids avoid straining when you go to the lavatory. Eat a diet high in fibre, as described in **Eating for a Perfect Pregnancy**, page 68. Follow the advice about psyllium husks in **Constipation**, page 140. You can apply witchhazel as a compress to help to reduce inflammation and soothe the area – leave it on for 20 minutes, three times a day. Alternatively, try comfrey or horse chestnut creams. After the pregnancy you may find that the haemorrhoids right themselves. Vitamin C rich foods, and a supplement of 1 g a day (with bioflavonoids) can help improve the connective tissue of the veins and thus prevent haemorrhoids in the first place. Bioflavonoids in foods are found in the natural bright colouring of fruit such as lemons, black grapes, plums, blackcurrants, apricots and rose hips. Vitamin E 400 ius daily and fish oils can help to ease blood flow. Rutin is a bioflavonoid available in capsules which helps to avoid and treat varicose veins and haemorrhoids

Exercise, such as walking and swimming, can help you to avoid varicose veins as they improve circulation. All the blood vessels go back up through one big vein in the groin and if this is compressed then pressure can build up in the legs below. At night elevate the mattress under your feet to encourage blood flow back up to your heart. As your bump gets bigger lie on your side for 20 minutes every few hours to relieve the pressure.

CHAPTER SEVEN

The Third Trimester

You are into the home straight now! Initially nine months probably seemed like an age, but now you will very soon be having your baby. Suddenly it all seems to have gone really quickly, and yet the last four weeks, as your bump becomes a bit more than any one wants to carry around, are likely to be a time when you can't wait to get on with the birth. Feelings of trepidation may be superseded by a sense of impatience as you look forward to meeting this little person that you have got to know so well. Even if you already know the sex of your baby, and think that you know if he or she is active or not, so many things about that little personality have yet to reveal themselves. What does your baby look like? Will your baby be lively or contemplative? Sleep a lot or be wakeful? How will you interact as a family? All will soon be revealed . . .

Now is not the time to let up with Eating for a Perfect Pregnancy. Your baby is growing fast and needs all the nourishment you can give. Babies deprived of nutrients in the last months of pregnancy tend to have larger heads and smaller abdomens, as the available nutrients are channelled into protecting the brain. This can lead to an increased risk of heart disease later in life, as the liver is less well developed. When you reach the last three months of your pregnancy you need to feed yourself and your baby better than ever to fuel the incredible spurt of growth that is about to happen.

WHAT IS HAPPENING TO YOU AND YOUR BABY

week 27 You should feel strong movements now as your baby's muscles are sufficiently developed to do somersaults. Your baby will push out against your stomach wall with hands and feet. You will probably have heard the baby's heartbeat by now on one of your antenatal visits. At 120–160 beats per minute it sounds incredibly fast, but the rate will slow down as it gets nearer to delivery time. The baby's skin is protected by a covering called the vernix, which keeps it supple and nourished.

week 28 Your baby is now about 36 cm/14 inches long and weighs over 900 g/2 lb. Your baby's hearing is becoming more acute and when your voice is recognised its heartbeat will speed up a little. Taste buds have now developed sufficiently for preferences to be instilled. If you have a liking for garlic, this taste will probably be transferred to the baby, and if you don't, the baby is likely to reject it. The brain develops most quickly from here on in and a large percentage of the brain cells that make up an adult brain are formed during this final period.

week 30 Back strain may become a problem as the uterus is now well above your belly button and your hormones have loosened your ligaments. Your baby's eyes are now learning to focus. You may not yet be aware of Braxton Hicks contractions ('rehearsal' contractions in readiness for the birth) but your baby probably is.

week 32 At about 1.8 kg/4 lb your baby has considerably less room to be active in the womb and he or she may even be moving into the head-down position. The lungs are maturing with the lining that prevents the air sacs collapsing after the birth now growing. Though perfectly formed, if your baby were born now it would still need an incubator.

week 34 As your baby kicks you can probably now make out the shape of a little hand or foot. Your baby is growing so quickly that you are putting on weight at a faster pace than before, and your blood volume has increased by 40 per cent. The baby can differentiate between light and dark and is bathed in a red glow when your tummy is in the sun.

week 36 Your baby should have now assumed a permanent head down position and weigh about 2.5–2.75 kg/5½–6 lb. This may feel strange with all that weight pressing down.

week 38 Your baby's weight is still increasing at a furious rate – as much as 25 g/1 oz a day. Eye movements and hand and feet reflexes are well co-ordinated and your baby is able to blink, turn its head towards a stimulus and seek milk.

week 40 Your baby is ready to be born and you are no doubt keen to meet the little person you've been nurturing for nine months. Ready, steady . . . GO!

week 41 Well you thought you were going to deliver on time, but junior isn't ready, so you have to do your beached whale impersonation for a little longer. Try not to get too frustrated as friends call you up to see if you have had your baby – they mean well! It won't be long now.

POSSIBLE CONCERNS IN THE THIRD TRIMESTER AND THEIR SOLUTIONS

Backache

Ten million women in the UK suffer from back pain, 80 per cent of them for more than a year. A job description that involves constantly lifting a struggling 6.8 kg/15 lb load would be considered highly suspect under government health in the workplace regulations. Yet all mothers have to contend with heavy toddlers, and the problems of backache often start in pregnancy.

As the baby grows, and your centre of gravity is pushed forwards, it is common to be affected by backache, especially if posture is poor and stomach muscles are not as strong as they could be. The softening and stretching of the stomach muscles (that normally support the back), which occurs as progesterone levels rise to prepare the muscles of the pelvic muscles for delivery, can make the situation worse. Paradoxically, if you suffer from back problems historically, this softening of the muscles can make chronic backache better for a while. The stomach muscles shorten after the birth, but unless you exercise them it is probably not enough to get them back into their pre-pregnancy state, and your back can be weakened in the long term. These are some of the things that you can do to address back problems:

● Check your posture and, if necessary, go to exercise classes that seek to remedy this problem.
● Avoid high heels as these destabilise the back muscles, and anyway a pregnant woman needs to be particularly poised to carry off balancing in high heels!
● Learn how to lift objects properly without straining your back. Rather than bending over from the waist, crouch down on your haunches.
● Learn how to get out of bed correctly by rolling on to your side, letting your legs drop over the edge of the bed, putting your weight on the arm nearest the mattress and levering yourself up using that arm. This avoids putting pressure on your back.
● Massage may help.
● Make sure your mattress is a good one.

● Drinking water, at least 2 litres/3½ pints daily, and avoiding dehydrating drinks such as alcohol, coffee and strong tea, helps to ensure that the muscles supporting your spine do not become dehydrated, which can diminish their effectiveness.

● Fish oils help to reduce inflammation; see also **The Natural Remedy Cupboard**, page 119, for herbs with pain relieving properties.

Heartburn

As many as 80 per cent of women experience heartburn in pregnancy. As the baby becomes larger, you may find that you suffer from reflux of the contents of your stomach, leaving an acidy feeling and taste. This is caused by the baby pressing on your stomach leaving little room for your food. The sphincter at the top of the stomach will be more relaxed because of the effects of progesterone levels, allowing reflux to occur. It can often be worse at night, making sleeping more difficult. To avoid heartburn eat smaller meals, more frequently, to give yourself the chance to digest them properly. Do not eat too late at night, and limit fluid with meals (but maintain fluid intake between meals). Spicy meals or fried food are likely to make the situation worse and you may be aware of foods that are triggers for you – coffee, acidic juices, bread, onions, meat, cheese, tomatoes, pastry. You may find relief by sleeping propped up with pillows, which allows gravity to help. Wear loose fitting clothes. Calcium based indigestion remedies are OK, but avoid aluminium based ones. Do not take indigestion remedies without first speaking to your doctor.

Herpes

Herpes simplex is a viral infection that is responsible for cold sores in the mouth and similar down below. It lies dormant in the infected area in between attacks, and while dormant does not present a problem. If you have a vaginal outbreak near the date of delivery, your obstetrician may consider a Caesarean to protect your baby against infection. Bolstering your immune system before and during pregnancy is the best way to reduce the severity and duration of any attacks. Keep all sugary and refined foods to a minimum, eat antioxidant rich foods (all fruit and vegetables) and increase foods in your diet that are rich sources of lysine. Lysine is an amino acid (protein building block) found in vegetables, sprouts, beans, fish, turkey, chicken, eggs, yoghurt, nutritional yeast, beef, milk and cheese. The way that lysine helps is by suppressing another amino acid, arginine, which actively promotes the herpes virus. Arginine rich foods to limit include nuts, seeds, wheat, rice, oats, raisins, chocolate, coffee, coconut, carob, aubergines, tomatoes, mushrooms and chickpeas. A daily dose of garlic can help to prevent and reduce the severity of outbreaks. Applying tea tree oil topically might help as it is anti-viral. A compound called resveratrol found naturally in red grapes and available as a supplement has been shown in one trial to significantly inhibit the herpes virus when applied topically to the affected area.

Insomnia

As your baby grows bigger you may find that the bulge makes it difficult for you to realign your position at night and get comfortable. Relaxation exercises can help. You can also get some relief by using pillows to prop yourself up in the night. If you are on your back, you may find it more comfortable to prop a pillow or two under your knees or, if you lie on your side, a pillow under one leg can help.

Sleeping remedies must not be taken without your doctor's say-so, this applies to herbal remedies too. Camomile tea is usually quite safe during pregnancy and can help to induce sleep and eating oat porridge late at night also seems to help (see **The Natural Remedy Cupboard**, page 119).

Itchy Skin

It is not uncommon for an itchy rash to appear under the breasts or in the groin. This can be because folds in the skin, created by increased weight, provide the opportunity for bacterial infections to develop. Wear loose cotton clothing, keep the area clean by washing with unperfumed soap, and apply calomine lotion. Tea tree oil or grapefruit seed extract, diluted in water, can help to keep any fungal infections at bay, but they must only be used externally and not taken internally. If your outbreak is eczema, piercing and rubbing on a capsule of evening primrose oil to the affected area twice daily can help to reduce the inflammation. Skin eruptions are not uncommon and are related to raging hormones. Itchy pimples, called puritic urticarial papules, can also develop, commonly in the same place as abdominal stretch marks. Vitamin C, 1 g daily, acts as an antihistamine and can help to reduce itchiness if you are susceptible to it.

If you develop a sudden rash-like reddening or generalised itching of the skin, particularly on your arms or legs, this may be a sign of obstetric cholestasis (your liver not working properly) and must be acted upon immediately. Your doctor will prescribe drugs to help bile flow, and early delivery may be necessary. If this condition is allowed to worsen it can lead to poisoning of the baby and a stillbirth.

Pelvic Floor Exercises

Sitting on the bus, or at work, you can quite happily and dutifully be doing your pelvic floor exercises and nobody need know! We are all aware of the importance of these exercises in keeping the muscles down below in shape and improving both the rate of your recovery from the birth and your sex life – but somehow they get forgotten about. Well it really is worth doing them, as all the evidence shows that they work. Some women also suffer from stress incontinence (urine leaks as a result of pressure or weakened muscles) and pelvic floor exercises help to avoid, or remedy, this. Several times a day, pull in the muscles of the area, as if you are stopping the flow of urine, and pull the muscles in all the way from the front to the back. Hold for a count of ten, release and then do ten quick pull-ins. Repeat three or four times to complete one session. Just for fun, and as a variation on the theme, use your vaginal muscles to write your name, shopping list, or as the originator of the idea suggested, Happy Birthday.

The best time to start these exercises is when you know you are pregnant, but if you have not already done so, then at least start them in your last trimester.

PREPARING FOR THE BIRTH

Many hours will be spent planning for the forthcoming event, in visiting your antenatal clinic weekly for a battery of checks, decorating the baby's room (with water based paints of course, and beware of glues and newly sawn chipboard as well) or buying in baby provisions.

In amongst all this activity take some time out to prepare your body for the delivery. Using the herbal tonics mentioned in **The Natural Remedy Cupboard** (see page 119) for the last couple of months of pregnancy is helpful to both tone and relax the uterine muscles. They also help you to stay relaxed and feel rested while you are in this pre-delivery phase.

Raspberry leaf is particularly well known for its applications in late pregnancy, but is also beneficial at the actual moment of birth. It has been used throughout history to encourage safe, easy births by helping to relax and tone the uterus. You can drink the tea for several weeks before the delivery (raspberry leaf tea bags are widely available from health food shops). It is equally effective to take raspberry leaf tablets when you go into labour. They are sold as a remedy for menstrual cramps, and will be marked 'not for use in pregnancy' as a caution, but you can ignore this if you are using them solely for when you go into labour. Start using the tablets as soon as you feel contractions, taking four (double the normal dose) every three hours. This short, intensive course should see you through the labour and help to ease the birth.

In the last three to four weeks of your pregnancy you may want to take 500 mg of evening primrose oil or blackcurrant seed oil, for the active compound GLA, as this can help boost your body's ability to make prostaglandins, which help to prepare the cervix for birth. If you find that you are overdue and your cervix is 'unripe' or not yet soft (which your midwife or doctor will be able to tell you upon examination) you can double the dose of GLA. As semen also contains these prostaglandins, you might also enjoy sex with your partner in late pregnancy (if it is comfortable, and as long as your doctor does not advise against it), as it may help to encourage labour.

There is also some evidence that women can help bring on labour if they stimulate their nipples for the grand total of 3 hours a day from the 39th week. The recommended procedure is to stimulate the nipples, areola (area around the nipples) and the breast with the balls of your fingertips, for 15 minutes per breast, alternating breasts for 1 hour in total. Do this three times per day. You can use creams and lotions and also rope in your partner, who may be only too willing. There is, however, also some risk that this will produce very strong contractions as it stimulates the hormone oxytocin. It certainly brings new meaning to twiddling your thumbs!

Part Four

NOW YOU ARE
A PARENT

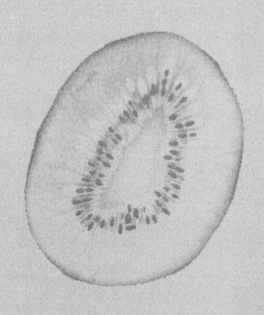

CHAPTER EIGHT

Now You Are a Parent

Your baby has arrived, and your experience of the actual birth will probably influence how you are feeling. You may find that you are living on a cloud of hormones which serve to pull you through the first few days. On the other hand, you may suffer a bout of postnatal depression, or be unusually uncomfortable after the birth. If you have had a vaginal birth your nether regions will be sore, ditto your tummy if you have had a Caesarean. This may be a dream-like time when night and day meld, and you bounce between euphoria and exhaustion. No amount of wise words, book scouring or holding of other people's babies will have prepared you for the impact of having a baby the first time round . . .

The experience is so different from woman to woman, and couple to couple, and of course some cope better than others. Whether or not there are worries attached to the baby's health also has a profound effect. I will not even try to go into the variables. What I want to focus on here are the things you can do to help yourself enjoy the experience as much as possible, and overcome the most obvious hurdles that may present themselves.

LOOKING AFTER YOU

Whatever the birth was like, easy or difficult, early or late, vaginal or Caesarean, accompanied by your partner or without, now is the time to really look after yourself so that you can bounce back as soon as possible. Much depends on your home circumstances, but only you can make yourself a priority at this time. So much attention is usually focused on the new arrival that the mother is frequently forgotten, as is the fact that she has to struggle with physical changes as well as the new baby. This means that she often needs to wave her hand above the crowd and say 'me too'.

We all know the stories about peasant women in rural cultures going off to have their baby in the midst of harvesting and then returning a couple of hours later, babe strapped on their backs, to resume their labours. I think just about every pregnant women has been regaled with this. But in all seriousness now is a time for physical recovery and rest, if you feel you need it, and you must not feel guilty taking more time out.

You may be experiencing an emotional explosion of intense love, or fear because you don't have these feelings. Hormones are all over the place – you are allowed to be a little irrational. Looking after a new baby, even if it sleeps a lot of the time initially, takes a huge chunk of time out of the day – especially if you've not done it before. Each fumbling nappy change seems to take for ever, each breast-feed takes half an hour, and just taking the baby out in the car can seem a major operation. Unless you are a very relaxed parent spontaneity seems to go out of the window. And don't forget, the average baby cries for about two hours a day in the first three months. But then there are loads of wonderful compensations.

Don't try to do it all yourself. Get some help from your partner, friends, grandparents or other family. There is no more selfish a being on this planet than a newborn baby, but that is as it should be – they have no other way of letting you know that they need something other than to cry, and as they are totally vulnerable we need to respond appropriately. Most parents manage to do this willingly, but even if you are a devoted angel of a parent, never forget that you have needs as well – it is OK to take time out as long as the baby is well catered for with someone you trust. You need time to promote your physical recovery, catch a couple of hours of sleep, exercise to get back into shape or just read a book and relax.

If you have a partner it may not be as difficult as you anticipate to get him to help. Men's testosterone levels crash by up to one-third after their baby is born, in a similar way to hormone changes in other species where the male does some of the nurturing. The lower his testosterone levels fall, the more the father dotes on his baby.

YOUR DIET WHILST BREAST-FEEDING

Many mothers express doubts about their ability to breast-feed, and whether they will have sufficient quantity of milk. In practice very few mothers are unable to breast-feed, it is more often a matter of overcoming problems with sore nipples.

From the point of view of the nutritional health of your baby, it is indisputably better to breast-feed than bottle feed, and it is also better to breast-feed for six months or more during the weaning period, rather than for a shorter period of time. Breast-feeding is protective from many points of view:

- Breast milk provides a perfect balance of nutrients.
- Antibodies in the milk help to protect against infections.
- Breast-feeding for a minimum of 13 weeks gives a baby increased protection against gastro-enteritis for up to 24 months.
- 15 weeks exclusive breast-feeding lowers the chance of respiratory problems such as asthma. There is also a reduced risk for the baby of eczema and ear or urinary infections.
- Breast milk contains special proteins that stimulate the

growth of several organs and the brain. There is evidence that breast-feeding is linked to improved brain function and intelligence probably because the balance of fats in breast milk.

- Extended breast-feeding, of at least nine months, is probably protective against susceptible children developing insulin dependent diabetes. It is believed that the cow's milk protein triggers an immune reaction in such children who are exposed at an early age.

From the mother's point of view there are also indisputable advantages:

- Convenience – no bottles to sterilise and wash. Economical too.
- Suckling induces sleepiness in the mother, making her more relaxed and improving night-time sleep.
- Breast-feeding encourages maternal weight loss – I always imagined that every pound the baby put on was another pound lost for the mother (this is not literally true, but it's as good a positive visualisation as any).
- It returns the uterus to its original size and shape by promoting the release of the hormone oxytocin.

One of the most frequently asked questions about breast-feeding is 'will I have enough milk?'. The answer is almost certainly yes. First of all, breast size does not determine the size of milk glands, and the average woman produces about 750 ml/27 fl oz of milk per day, which is equivalent to around 500 calories for the baby. The easiest way to tell if you are producing sufficient milk, and whether your baby is getting enough to be satisfied, is if your baby is putting on weight. If the baby's weight is increasing at a satisfactory rate, you are providing ample milk for his or her needs. Again, one of the most important factors that will determine the quantity, as well as the quality, of your milk is how well nourished you are and how supportive your diet is of your health while you are breast-feeding.

While breast-feeding you need around 500 calories more than you would do normally. During the first three months alone your baby will double his or her birth weight – and it all comes just from you. By following the Eating for a Perfect Pregnancy regime you will fulfill your nutritional needs. You also need to maintain your fluid intake and drink maybe a bit more than normal, as producing milk uses up so much liquid. If you do not do this you run an increased risk of eczema and other dry skin complaints and constipation. Instead of the normal 2 litres/3½ pints of water a day, be prepared to drink around 3 litres/5¼ pints to avoid drying up like a prune. Contrary to popular belief, you do not need to drink milk to make milk. What you do need to do is to ensure that you are still getting sufficient calcium levels in your diet to meet the requirements of a rapidly growing baby. It is also desirable to maintain sufficient iron and zinc levels in your diet to avoid becoming depleted, as your milk passes nutrients along to your baby. Essential fats continue to be vitally important and eczema (on you or your baby) is a sign that you may not be getting enough. If this is the case, slightly increase the amount of flax oil you are taking daily until the eczema disappears. One or two table-spoons a day is sufficient for most people.

There are only three potential problems with breast-feeding, from the nutritional point of view, which must be considered. Of course there are many other possible issues, such as the mother's emotional feelings about it, but again I must leave those to other books and concentrate solely on the nutritional aspects.

The three possible issues are:

- The quality of the milk, and therefore the mother's ability to nurture her child with breast-feeding, depends on the quality of the mother's diet. If there are insufficient nutrients in the mother's diet, the baby will not be getting the best out of being breast-fed.

- There is now plenty of evidence that breast milk is contaminated with around 350 pollutants such as dioxins and PCBs. Even the milk of breast-feeding Inuit mothers, who are about as far away from pollution as it is possible to be, is contaminated to a high level because of pollution drifting across the world. There is a health anomaly here because one of the few ways that a woman can get rid of these pollutants, which are fairly insoluble and reside in the body without being excreted, is to breast-feed. What a dilemma. The hugely difficult question to answer is: is it still better to breast-feed even though the baby may be receiving a dose of chemical pollutants? There is probably no straightforward answer to this, as it is too new a problem to analyse and understand all the associated issues. On balance, I would say that the benefits of breast-feeding still outweigh the negative effects that these pollutants are likely to have on the baby. Formula milk can be equally contaminated and does not have the advantages of breast milk, such as building up the baby's immune system. The mother can make sure that she minimises her contact with chemicals by eating organic food, drinking filtered water, and not allowing the food she eats to come into contact with plastics.

- Some mothers, for example those that have a medical condition that might impact on the baby, are simply unable to breast-feed. If the mother is HIV positive, if she is epileptic or if she is on medication which is contra-indicated for the baby while breast-feeding, she might need to bottle feed. Supporting your general health is one of the best ways of ensuring that you do not get infections which might need medicating. If you find that you need to take antibiotics while breast-feeding, and the doctor says it is safe to carry on breast-feeding, you can protect your baby by giving him or her some baby formulated probiotics (beneficial bacteria) such as bifido infantis (see **Resources**, page 197).

What to Avoid Whilst You Are Breast-feeding

The list is pretty much the same as when you are pregnant, as it is important to avoid drugs that can be passed along to the baby. If you have resumed coffee and tea drinking and you find that your baby is not sleeping properly, don't be too surprised – the caffeine can affect your baby through your breast milk and act as a stimulant. You can re-introduce some foods that you have been avoiding back into your diet, but as you will still want to keep infections at bay to avoid having to take antibiotics you will need to make sure that your suppliers are reliable, that the produce is very fresh and that your food preparation methods are scrupulous.

The culinary herb sage, if used in largish amounts, can reduce milk flow, as can vitamin B6, which you should not take in excess of more than 50 mg daily.

You must not use the combined oestrogen-progestogen contraceptive pill when breast-feeding, as it can influence both the quantity and the quality of the milk, and affect the baby. If you want to use the Pill at all (and you may prefer to use natural or barrier contraception methods), it is best to use the progestogen-only Pill, or mini-Pill, which can be prescribed during breast-feeding.

POSSIBLE CONCERNS AFTER YOUR BABY IS BORN

After a Caesarean

Whether you have had a Caesarean as an elective procedure or as an emergency procedure, it is still important to recognise that it is major surgery and you must allow yourself six to eight weeks to get over it. Of course, doing this while you are juggling a little baby is no mean feat. Caesareans are on the increase, from one in ten in 1985 to one in eight or one in five, depending on the hospital, today. The nutrients that promote healing of tissues are vitamin C, zinc and essential fats. Taking the homeopathic remedy, arnica, can reduce bruising. Piercing a vitamin E capsule and gently rubbing the contents on to the scar can help to promote healing, and again zinc and vitamin C cream can be beneficial (see **Resources**, page 197). While you must not take the herb comfrey internally, it can be used safely as a poultice. Its common name, 'knitbone', is an indication of how useful it is at helping to repair damaged tissues. If you do not have access to any fresh comfrey leaves you can buy them dried or as tea bags. Steep them in water and apply as a poultice to the scar tissue.

Cot Death – Minimising the Risks

Each year in the UK 350 babies die of sudden infant death syndrome. The devastation of cot death is something that every parent dreads, and the grief for a parent who suffers the loss of a baby dying from such a tragedy can only be guessed at. Why do so many apparently healthy babies die suddenly in their sleep? We don't yet know the answer, but there are a number of factors that have been linked to these tragedies. Respiratory problems, in particular, have been closely linked to cot death, which is why parental smoking and overheating the baby are to be avoided. Here is a checklist of the most important consider-ations and the steps you can take to lessen the risk:

- Lie the baby on its back to sleep as this has been linked to a tenfold reduction in risk.
- Give up smoking and certainly do not allow your baby to be regularly exposed to cigarette smoke. Even if you smoke out of the room, do not approach the baby within 15–30 minutes of smoking.
- Your baby should sleep in a room temperature of about 65F. Avoid the risk of the blanket going over the head by tucking your baby in at the bottom end of the mattress. Do not use duvets, hot water bottles or electric blankets. As long as the cot mattress is well aired and easy to clean, there is no evidence of one type of mattress being an improvement on any other.
- High maternal intake of caffeine during pregnancy has been linked to cot death in some studies.
- There is a suspicion that allergy may be at the root of some cot deaths. High levels of the enzyme tryptase, a unique component of lung mast cells (which react to allergies), have sometimes been observed. If your family tends towards allergies (asthma, hay fever, eczema, psoriasis) then possibly be cautious about using formula milk instead of breast-feeding, as cow's milk allergy is one of the most common allergies.
- If you are breast-feeding, take 1 g of vitamin C daily, the benefit of which will pass through in your breast milk.
- Very early research has found an 80 per cent link between helicobacter pylori stomach infection and cot death. Good hand hygeine and breast feeding are the best ways to reduce this possible risk.

Healing Your Nether Regions

Two thirds of vaginal births result in tears or episiotomies (surgical cutting to enlarge the perineum) and some mothers may feel afterwards that they have more stitches in them than a hand-made Dior dress. To improve comfort and healing time there are several things you can do. First and foremost are you still doing your pelvic floor exercises? They help. Make sure that you are getting enough fibre in your diet to help with going to the lavatory – the last thing you need to be doing when you have all those stitches is to be straining. If your bowel movements are less than ideal, then now is the time to employ the services of psyllium husks (see **Constipation**, page 140), and make sure, too, that you are religiously drinking enough water and avoiding dehydrating drinks. Take care that your vitamin C and zinc levels are good, as they are vital for repair of wounds. Take a tablespoon of flax oil daily on your food to provide essential fats, as they also speed up healing. Taking the homeopathic remedy arnica can reduce bruising, and this will also pass into your breast milk to help your baby get over the birth.

No Sex Please (We're Parents)

Your midwife or doctor will talk to you about contraception about six weeks after the birth, as if sex were a serious possibility! Lack of sleep, physical discomfort from healing stitches and a routine that is turned completely upside down will stymie even the best sex lives. No doubt some people do have a stab at it (pun intended), but many will then retire to their separate corners and not repeat the experiment for a while. Do not feel that you are somehow deficient if this corresponds with what you are experiencing, those who say that they resumed an active and imaginative sex life in the first few months are either in the minority or being economical with the truth. Forty per cent of women say they have a very low libido three months after the birth. Take time to let your sex life resume, otherwise any stress linked to this will compound other stresses and insecurities. When the time is right, both of you will know. In the meantime, keep doing your pelvic floor exercises and support yourself nutritionally to maximise your energy levels in readiness for all the fun to come.

Postnatal Depression

Nobody really knows why 5–10 per cent of mothers are affected by postnatal depression, and it is most likely to be multi-factorial. It is important to deal with this problem as early as possible because affected mothers can find it more difficult to relate well to their babies. What is certain is that nutrition can have quite a lot to do with it, and a well-nourished mother is less likely to be affected. In particular, zinc levels are important, which is logical given that this mineral is so important for correct brain functioning. Other brain nurturing nutrients that are important include B-vitamins and essential fats (see pages 85 and 53 for food sources of these).

Maintaining magnesium and calcium levels is also important to offset postnatal depression. It comes as no surprise to learn that when babies are more irritable than normal mothers are more likely to suffer from postnatal depression. If your baby is particularly irritable you may want to investigate whether he or she has colic. This may be brought on by substances you are eating that are coming through in your breast milk. The most common foods for this are the garlic and onion family and wheat and dairy products. Following through the theme of maternal stress or anxiety, if a mother has good support at home from a partner or from family she is less likely to suffer. If you can say 'take the baby off my hands while I have a bath', there is obviously less pressure and more time to preserve energy levels and regenerate after the birth. If the mother is denied this opportunity it will inevitably lead to a greater drain on her nutrient reserves as stress kicks in and greedily uses up nutrients. There is good evidence that mothers who give their babies regular baby massage have less postnatal depression, perhaps because of the bonding process, or perhaps because it just relaxes the mother and reduces stress. Baby massage also helps babies with trapped wind and colic (especially tummy massage in gentle, circular, clockwise movements). Many health authorities now offer classes in baby massage to new mothers.

Sore Nipples and Breast Engorgement

Sore nipples are no joke. After several days of having a baby's jaws firmly clamped to your nipples, they usually protest. Many mothers go through a phase where they almost can't bear to breast-feed because it is just too painful. It is rather a shame that sore and cracked nipples are among the main reasons why mothers give up breast-feeding, to the detriment of their child's long-term health. If your nipples are cracking, piercing a vitamin E capsule and rubbing it on to the area can be a tremendous help, soothing, lubricating and helping to heal the tissue. Sore nipples and engorged breasts are also helped by putting a dark green cabbage leaf on each breast and letting the enzymes in the cabbage exert their healing effect on the breast tissue. Bruise the cabbage leaves first to release more enzymes, and store in the refrigerator so they are also delightfully cooling. When you are cringing with discomfort as your baby feeds you may find it difficult to believe that it will ever get better, but your nipples do toughen up quite quickly and if you can work through this uncomfortable phase, the rest is usually plain sailing. A flannel soaked in very cold water, or an ice pack (frozen peas in their packet) can all help engorged breast discomfort. To relieve engorgement feed regularly (even if you have to wake the baby), and express a little milk first so that your baby can latch on to the flattened nipples. Again, this problem will pass if you persevere. Mastitis is when an infection sets in in the breasts and antibiotics are prescribed to relieve this.

Too Tired to Tango

The most common postnatal complaint is tiredness. This is no wonder, as most mothers lose 400–600 hours of sleep in the first year of a baby's life. And goodness knows what the statistics are for a mother with a toddler and a new baby as well.

For all the benefits of breast-feeding, it is important to realise that it uses up a lot of energy. This is not a reason to give up breast-feeding, but it is something to acknowledge in order that you do not run yourself ragged. Apart from giving yourself plenty of time to rest, the most important thing is to keep Eating for a Perfect Pregnancy (or in this case Eating for Motherhood). If you are unnaturally tired, and are also more pale than usual, you may want to get your doctor to check if you are anaemic. Blood loss, as well as an extra call on your reserves, may have tipped the balance of your iron levels. Apart from iron, the nutrients needed for energy production are the B-vitamins, vitamin C and magnesium, so make sure you eat foods that are rich in these nutrients. Even if you are keen to lose weight, do not diet yet. If you are bottle feeding you are likely to struggle a bit more to lose a few extra pounds than if you are breast-feeding. Nevertheless, you still need nutrients to heal, avoid tiredness and build up reserves depleted by pregnancy. If you are not stabilising your weight when eating sensibly then you probably need to increase your activity levels and exercise.

While you are breast-feeding you still need to apply the principle of Eating for a Perfect Pregnancy as your baby needs all those nutrients, and so do you. In any event, if you are breast-feeding this will help to strip off the excess weight.

It may seem improbable while you are still getting used to your new baby-centred schedule, but if you can resume exercise six weeks after having your baby this will help to boost energy levels. If you do manage to exercise remember to include some tummy toners to strengthen your back in readiness for weight-lifting a small child.

GROWING A HEALTHY CHILD

You have worked at giving your baby the best possible start in life you can by addressing your diet. Now is the time to resolve to continue your good work and make sure that the positive changes you have made are for life, for yourself and for your whole family. When you begin to feed your baby have just one guiding principle – this is the most precious little person, so give him or her only the best quality food that you are able. The principles are the same as those I have been emphasising throughout this book – stick to energy enhancing and nutrient dense foods that are unadulterated by chemicals. For information on how to go about this, and on weaning and first foods, read my book *What Should I Feed My Baby?*.

Part Five

RESOURCES

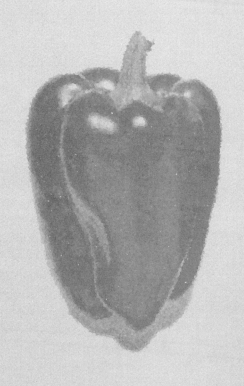

To find out more about Suzannah Olivier's activities see her website at: www.healthandnutrition.co.uk. email: eattobefit@aol.com

HERBAL AND NUTRIENT SUPPLEMENT SUPPLIERS

BIOCARE Birmingham Tel: 0121 433 3727

Stocked by good independent health food shops.
● nutrients: large range of vitamins, minerals and essential fats
● preconception/pregnancy formula: antenatal plus (women), ASC (men)
● baby formulated beneficial bacteria (bifob infantis)

BLACKMORES

Available from good quality health food shops. A full range of good quality herbs and nutrients for every need.

HEALTH PLUS East Sussex Tel: 01323 492096

● nutrients: range of nutrients available in convenient daily dose packs – each contains a combination of supplements that are designed for specific health conditions
● preconception/pregnancy formula: pregnancy pack (one month's supply of 28 daily packs)

HIGHER NATURE East Sussex Tel: 01435 882880

Direct mail ordering service available.
● nutrients: range of vitamins, minerals and essential fats; they also supply flaxseed oil and essential balance oil, which are an excellent alternative to other salad oils

LAMBERTS Kent Tel: 01892 552120

Available from good independent health food retailers.
● nutrients: large range of vitamins, minerals and essential fats

NUTRI LTD High Peak Tel: 0800 212742

● nutrients: a comprehensive range of vitamins, minerals and essential fats
● preconception/pregnancy formulas: Prenatal phase 1, Prenatal phase 2, Prenatal phase 3

THE NUTRI CENTRE London WI Tel: 020 7436 5122

Stock an extensive range of nutrition products, health foods and books
from various suppliers and manufacturers. They also have their own
range, NutriWest. You can visit the shop and all their stock is available
by mail order.

SOLGAR Herts Tel: 01442 890355 www.solgar.com

Stocked by good independent health food shops.

● nutrients: a large range of low to high dose vitamins, minerals and
essential fats

● preconception/pregnancy formula: prenatal nutrients

FORESIGHT

Pre-conceptual Care Range of nutrients designed by Foresight (see **Support Services**, page 199).

VITABIOTICS

Pregnacare
Available from most large chemists.

GNC (GENERAL NUTRITON CENTRE) www.gnc.com

GNC Prenatal Formula
Available from national GNC health food shop chain.

FINDING A THERAPIST

BRITISH ASSOCIATION OF NUTRITIONAL
THERAPISTS (BCM BANT) London WCIN 3XX Tel: 0870 6061284

For a list of registered nutrition therapists please send a large SAE to BANT
at the above address.

INSTITUTE FOR OPTIMUM NUTRITION (ION)

Blades Court Deodar Road London SW15 2NU Tel: 020 8877 9993
Call for a directory of nutritionists.

BRITISH SOCIETY FOR ALLERGY, ENVIRONMENTAL AND
NUTRITIONAL MEDICINE (BSAENM) Southampton Tel: 01703
812 124

For a list of medical doctors who have a particular interest in nutritional
medicine.

**SOCIETY FOR THE PROMOTION OF NUTRITIONAL
THERAPY** PO Box 626 Woking GU22 OXD Tel: 01483 740 903
For information, please send an SAE and £1 to the above address.

THE BRITISH HERBAL MEDICINE ASSOCIATION
Tel: 01453 751 389
To obtain details of a qualified herbal practitioner in your area.

SUPPORT SERVICES

FORESIGHT 28 The Paddock Godalming Surrey GU7 1XD
Tel: 01483 427839
Organisation for pre-conceptual care.

FAMILY PLANNING ASSOCIATION (FPA) Tel: 020 7837 4044
To find a natural family planning teacher.

ZITA WEST PREGNANCY PRODUCTS Tel: 08701 668899
Mail order.

ORGANIC FOOD SOURCES

THE SOIL ASSOCIATION 86 Colston Street Bristol BS1 5BB
Tel: 0117 929 0661
The Soil Association can provide a list of organic suppliers in the UK, as
well as publications on organic issues. Telephone to check the price of
the catalogue.

SIMPLY ORGANIC Tel: 0845 1000 444 www.simplyorganic.net
Nationwide delivery of organic food.

WATER DISTILLER SUPPLIERS

WHOLISTIC RESEARCH COMPANY
Tel: 01954 781074

HIGHER NATURE
Tel: 01435 882880

AQUAPURE DISTILLATION
Tel: 020 8892 9010

FRESHWATER FILTER COMPANY
Tel: 020 8558 7495

THE FRESHWATER COMPANY
Tel: 0345 023998
Delivery service of pre-distilled water in the South East of England.

BOOKS

What Should I Feed My Baby? Suzannah Olivier (Weidenfield & Nicholson, 1998)

Postnatal Exercise Book Margie Polden and Barbara Whiteford (Frances Lincoln, 1992)

What To Expect When You're Expecting Arlene Eisenberg, Heidi Murkoff and Sandee Hathaway (Simon & Schuster, 1996)

The New Pregnancy and Childbirth Sheila Kitzinger (Penguin, 1997)